The How-To of Psychotherapy

This is an essential guide for therapists at the beginning of their career. It goes beyond academic theory to provide readers with confidence and competence around core aspects of therapeutic processes, so they can contend with professional and ethical issues as well as assist in establishing their identity and standing as a therapist.

Informed by years of clinical work and supervision, Bianca Denny presents practical answers to burning questions in an authoritative and accessible manner. The book offers plain language explanations of common dilemmas that often flummox trainee and early-career therapists, such as keeping time in session, coping with "imposter syndrome", decisions around managing confidentiality, and working with patients who get under your skin. These are accompanied by practical tips and ready-to-implement skills, encouraging readers to consider the application of these skills to the patients and presentations in their current practice. Further supported by diagrams, tables, and call-out boxes, the book is easy to navigate and revisit throughout the first weeks, months, and years of a career in psychotherapy.

Practical and accessible, this book is ideal for trainee and early-career psychologists, psychotherapists, counsellors, social workers, and other helping professionals.

Bianca Denny (D.Psych) is a clinical psychologist, working in private practice in Melbourne, Australia. She is an accredited supervisor of trainee (provisional) psychologists and those seeking clinical endorsement. Bianca also contributes to the media, writing on mental health and psychology topics.

The How-To of Psychotherapy

A Practical Guide for Therapists

BIANCA DENNY

Routledge
Taylor & Francis Group

LONDON AND NEW YORK

Designed cover image: Getty Images

First published 2026
by Routledge
4 Park Square, Milton Park, Abingdon, Oxon OX14 4RN

and by Routledge
605 Third Avenue, New York, NY 10158

Routledge is an imprint of the Taylor & Francis Group, an informa business

British Library Cataloguing-in-Publication Data
A catalogue record for this book is available from the British Library

ISBN: 978-1-032-87516-3 (hbk)
ISBN: 978-1-032-87515-6 (pbk)
ISBN: 978-1-003-53303-0 (ebk)

DOI: 10.4324/9781003533030

Typeset in Dante and Avenir
by Apex CoVantage, LLC

Contents

Acknowledgements

I am indebted to my own therapists and supervisors. And also to my patients, who are always the greatest teachers any therapist can have.

Special thanks to the therapists whose experiences and "words of wisdom" are integrated throughout this book: Laura Baldwin, Laura Beddoe, Amanda Bolton, Joanne Burch, Andrew Francis, Marcelle Gray, Elisabeth Hanscombe, Cat Kirby, Larissa McKay, Amanda Murtagh, Selma Music, Stephanie Perin, Mayumi Purvis, Matthew Roberts, Phoebe Rogers, Carol Sandiford, Monique Slevison, Ruby Swaid, Andrew Telley, and David Young.

Introduction

1

Every therapist was once a beginner.

Sigmund Freud. Nancy McWilliams. Aaron Beck. Judith Beck. Marcia Linehan. Irvin Yalom. Carl Rogers. Rollo May. John and Julie Gottman. Melanie Klein. Peter Levine. Jeffrey Young. Esther Perel.

Giants of psychotherapy, renowned and revered. These celebrated therapists were all once at the beginning of their tenure, just as you are now.

The beginnings of a career in the helping professions will look different for each person. Therapists come in all shapes and forms – varied gender, age, race, culture, and socio-economic backgrounds. Professional affiliations and training backgrounds may include social work, psychology, counselling, occupational therapy, medicine, nursing, psychiatry, and chaplaincy. Therapeutic modalities and the work of each individual differs greatly within and between each of these professional groups. Regardless, all therapists are tied together by a central and common aim: the use of talking therapy to assist with psychological well-being.

★★

The how-to of psychotherapy

This book was borne of my own experiences of training and working as a therapist. Working with supervisees – from trainees through to established therapists – highlighted the need for an accessible and timely resource to assist therapists to answer many of the vexing questions that arise from this challenging but rewarding profession.

DOI: 10.4324/9781003533030-1

The structure and format of this book is informed by the information and knowledge acquired from more than a decade of providing supervision to trainee and early-career therapists. Time and time again, supervisees express similar questions and quandaries, usually prefaced with, "I know this sounds stupid, but . . .":

- I always run over time in session.
- How can I encourage a reluctant patient to speak?
- I cannot sit with any silence in session. It feels awkward, so I rush to speak to fill the space.
- My patient is not improving, I must be doing something wrong.
- My patient disengaged. What did I do wrong?
- What happens if I see my patient in a social setting, outside of the consulting room?
- I am always behind on my notes and paperwork.
- I am spending evenings and weekends catching up on my notes and paperwork, and I still feel behind.
- How can I overcome my "imposter syndrome"?
- My colleagues seem to know so much more than me.
- A particular patient is really getting under my skin. I don't think I can work with them any longer.
- I am worried that I disclosed personal information about myself to a patient. Where do I go from here?
- My patient disclosed something that I think might need to be reported to an authority. I am worried this will impact our therapeutic relationship.
- I'm thinking about going into private practice. What are the pros and cons?
- I feel completely burnt out. But my patients need me, so there's no way I can schedule a break.
- Being a therapist is tough. I don't think I'm cut out for it. I am re-thinking my decision to work in this field.

My story

I share a brief overview of my experience of becoming a therapist here, in the hope that it will demonstrate the many pathways to training and working as a therapist. Setbacks are normal and experienced by most people who aspire to work as a therapist. The training is challenging in various ways, but it is also rewarding and worthwhile. The profession itself offers diversity and flexibility.

Similar to most therapists, my own pathway to this profession featured a few twists and turns. In retrospect, I wanted to be a therapist before I had acquired the language or cognitive capacity to know such a job existed. From an early age, I had an interest in people and their behaviour. I was a quiet child, prone to obstinance and observation. My natural propensity to gathering and analysing information complemented a growing curiosity about what I now understand to be "the human condition" – how to make sense of the unique ways that people think, feel, and behave.

My interest in human behaviour would lead me to performing what I would now recognise as early attempts to conduct experiments. Noticing a behaviour or trend, making an observation, collecting information or data, and then evaluating results. I applied this thinking to all sorts of matters – how often we ate the same family dinner at home (often), how many cars on the road were white (many), whether males or females did more domestic labour (the latter).

Later, during my high school years, I realised there was a name for my interest in human behaviour – psychology. Imagine my delight when I realised not only was this a legitimate area of study, but it also offered career prospects.

I was excited to study psychology in the senior years of secondary school, seeing it as a stepping stone to tertiary studies and employment in the field. Having found "hard sciences" such as biology and chemistry unappealing, psychology offered a more palatable foray into study. I had found my niche.

Conducting a classic experiment in which we tested Jean Piaget's development stages (sensorimotor, pre-operational, concrete operational, and formal operational) represented a seminal moment in my learning and firmly ensconced my ambition to further pursue psychology studies.

At university I enrolled in psychology. My determined plan to complete the training pathway required for registration as a psychologist as efficiently as possible fell apart somewhere through the first semester of study. Like many undergraduate psychology students, I struggled with statistics and found the introductory psychology subjects more than a little dry. Similar to many university students, I felt overwhelmed by the jump from high school to university; suddenly, I was a very small fish in a very big pond. I was easily distracted from study by burgeoning social opportunities. New friendships and off-campus activities offered a welcome reprieve from the demands of assignments and exams.

Imposter syndrome in full flight, my trepidation was not aided by the lecturer's assertion in our first class; in a seemingly well-rehearsed act, he instructed us to look around the overcrowded theatre (such was the popularity of undergraduate psychology courses that students were literally sitting in the aisles and blocking doorways), asking how many students planned to work as therapists. A cascade of hands shot up, like a lecture theatre version of a Mexican Wave. It seemed even eagerness was a point of competition among students. The lecturer laughed in a manner that can only be described as a chortle, telling us admonishingly that just a handful of the hundreds of students would complete the studies necessary to work in the field. I would later recognise the lecturer's charade as an act of Schadenfrëude (a German phrase for taking pleasure or deriving satisfaction from another's misfortune).

He was right. Along with many others in my cohort, I soon dropped my psychology subjects, opting instead to major in history. After graduation, I shirked an offer for further history studies in favour of a prolonged overseas working holiday.

I returned to my home country a few years later. A little older, a lot wiser, and ready to concentrate on pursuing further study. Upon reflection, living and working overseas was excellent preparation for working as a therapist. My world became bigger, both figuratively and metaphorically. Overseas, I was an even smaller fish in an even bigger pond. I learned about people, their lives, their misfortunes, their joys, their losses, their assumptions, their ideals, and their ideas. I had fun, took risks, made mistakes, navigated unknown terrain, and had my own core beliefs about myself and the world challenged. My perspective on the world was no longer the only one I considered. I felt better equipped to understand therapy, from both a theoretical and an applied position.

Back on home soil, I was once again a psychology student. In my late 20s, I epitomised the bookish life of a "mature age student"; a conscientious learner, seated in the front row of the lecture theatre. This time around, I was not intimidated by statistics, nor bored by the theory-laden introductory psychology subjects.

Then, a trainee therapist.[1] After completing the sequence of undergraduate psychology subjects required to enter postgraduate study, I undertook a doctoral degree in clinical psychology. The three-year degree featured three integrated components: coursework (including lectures and assignments), internships (including 200 days of face-to-face patient contact), and an 80,000-word research thesis.

Then, an early-career therapist. I commenced part-time work at a community health service while completing a postdoctoral research fellowship. Juggling academic work and the demands of a growing young family, I began work in private practice under the supervision and guidance of an experienced therapist. Eventually, I established my own private practice.

Later, I gained qualifications in specific modalities, expanding upon cognitive behaviour therapy (CBT) and acceptance and commitment therapy (ACT), which formed the basis of much of my training and early-career work. I became accredited as a supervisor, overseeing the work of trainee therapists and providing supervision to therapists seeking general guidance and those pursuing endorsement in the area of clinical psychology.

Along the way, I expanded from clinical practice. Indulging my passion for research and reading, I looked beyond one-on-one therapy work to include non-therapy roles. This included conference presentations, convening workshops and seminars, publishing research articles in peer-reviewed journals, contributing to book chapters, authoring a book, and writing for media outlets. This diversification has helped make my role as a therapist viable and sustainable.

What is therapy?

There is much more to therapy than the time spent face-to-face with a patient during a therapy session. Just like an iceberg (see Figure 1.1), most

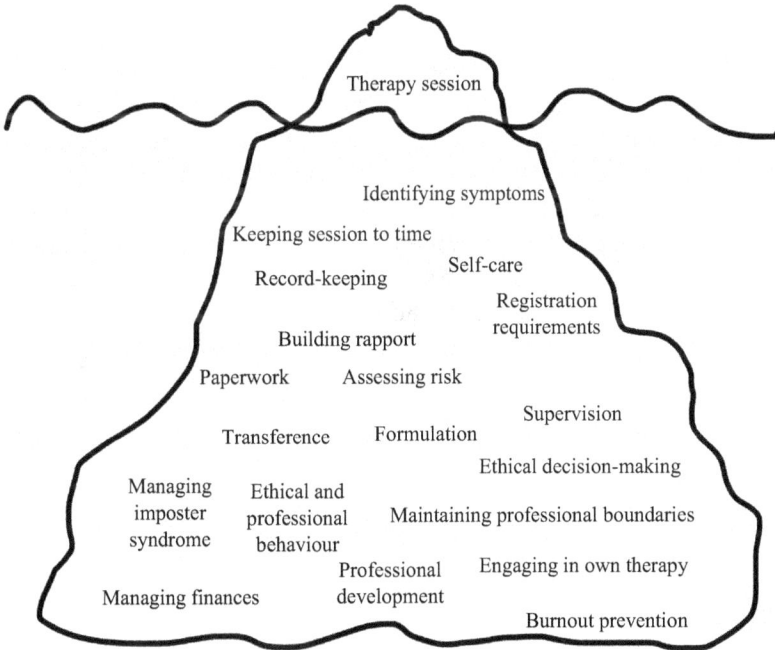

Figure 1.1 Factors relevant to talking therapy.

activity happens out of sight. Underneath the surface, the "conversation" between a therapist and patient is underpinned by a flurry of planning, activity, thought, and clinical skill.

Learning the craft of therapy is similar to acquiring any new skill. Take, for example, driving a motor vehicle. Novice drivers focus (and often hyper-focus) on the basics – accelerating, braking, memorising traffic rules. They are often hypervigilant of other cars, worried about what other drivers may be thinking of them, and avoidant of any manoeuvre deemed difficult, such as parallel parking or merging with traffic. But one day, usually without any fanfare or warning, these skills become second nature. Few drivers can pinpoint the moment of transition from novice to experienced driver. Eventually, everything clicks.

Similarly, few therapists can pinpoint the moment of transition from being a novice to an experienced and a competent therapist. Such is the ordinariness of this extraordinary development that this transition remains hidden in the milieu of therapeutic work; somewhere along the way, the micro-skills and macro-skills inherent to therapy became second nature. Just like driving a car. Therapists (and drivers) may be unsure of exactly what lies ahead, but with the right support, all novice therapists can develop the confidence and competence to manage what may come.

Therapist development

The trajectory of becoming a therapist is conceptualised here as encompassing three overlapping stages. First, the *trainee* therapist. Second, the *early-career* therapist. And last, the *established* therapist (see Figure 1.2).

The vocation of being a therapist provides a secure, long-term career. There is no rush to learn everything. For most therapists, learning their trade is lifelong. Becoming an established therapist is a continuous process. For trainees and early-career therapists, the goal is to gain a thorough understanding of the theoretical basis of talk therapy and master foundational therapeutic skills. The rest will come with time and practice.

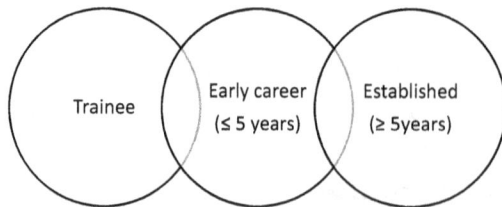

Figure 1.2 Therapist developmental stages.

Research indicates increased demand for therapy services in recent years. Psychological distress associated with events such as the COVID-19 pandemic and a seemingly increased sense of global distress around issues such as climate change and geopolitical crises has precipitated high demand for therapy services. Better understanding of mental illness and improved community awareness of mental health and mental illness has promoted a more open dialogue about therapy and its benefits, leading to a greater acceptance of being "in therapy". Therapy-speak has entered the cultural vernacular; terms (such as, anxiety, depression, burnout) that were previously in the domain of mental health professionals are now common parlance (Denny, 2023). Mental health is being de-mystified and de-stigmatised, prompting more people than ever to seek professional support.

Theories of therapist development

Much research in the area of therapist training and development seeks to answer the oft-asked question: what makes a good therapist? To this end, several theories and models have been proposed. Common to each are factors thought relevant to the path from trainee to established therapist, including innate interpersonal skills, a propensity towards helping others, and attunement to patients' cues and needs over time. Each theory points to therapy skills becoming increasingly sophisticated and integrated over time.

Rønnestad and Skovholt (2003) proposed a six-stage model of therapist development (see Figure 1.3). The altruistic and interpersonal skills

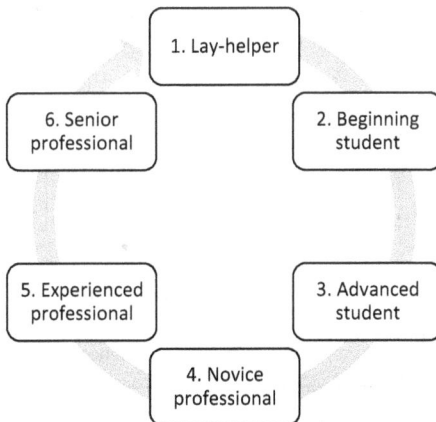

Figure 1.3 Rønnestad and Skovholt's (2003) stages of therapist development.

necessary to becoming an effective therapist are theorised to be innate and present in the early years of life, predisposing individuals to pursue work as a helping professional, such as being a therapist. The beginner and student phases are followed by being a novice professional. The stage of novice professional is typically considered to be the first few years following graduation or obtainment of license to practise as a therapist. Experienced professionals have practised for several years, while therapists in the senior professional phase are well-established and regarded by others as senior.

In its simplest form, this model presents a linear progression through the career stages of being a therapist. However, similar to the learning of any skill, progress over time may wax and wane. An "experienced professional" may revert to a "novice professional" when, for example, commencing training in a new therapeutic modality or working with a patient with a novel presentation.

This model reinforces the notion of therapists as lifelong learners. Years of experience can bring seniority and wisdom, but no therapist can be an expert in everything, no matter how many years of practice or how many hundreds of patients. Good therapists acknowledge their strengths while also recognising knowledge deficits and areas of relative weakness.

Similar to Rønnestad and Skovholt's (2003) model, Hogan's classic model of therapist development posits the building of autonomy and confidence over time (Reising & Daniels, 1983). This is an important model for trainee and early-career therapists to note, as it demonstrates expectations regarding capacity to work independently. As seen in Figure 1.4, closer supervision is required in the early stages of training and work as a therapist. Over time, this gives way to self-competence that allows the therapist to work with increased independence and creativity.

Therapist development has also been likened to the maternal experience (Clarke, 2010). With reference to Donald Winnicott, the renowned English

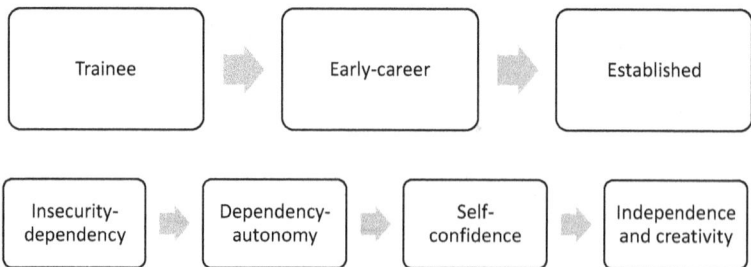

Figure 1.4 Typical trajectory of therapist development.

paediatrician and psychoanalyst known for his influential work in perinatal mental health, Clarke (2010) proposed that over time therapists learn to understand patients' cues in order to better understand their needs, just as mothers learn to understand their baby's cues (such as crying) to meet the infant's needs. Both roles – that of therapist and mother – are assisted by a foundation of intellectual knowledge, but demand much on-the-job-learning. As any senior therapist or parent will tell a budding therapist or expectant mother, respectively, "You don't yet know what you don't yet know". Therapist training is a developmental experience; sensitivities, skills, and confidence grow over time.

Two major schools of thought pervade training programmes. The first perspective proposes that trainee therapists enter into training programmes as "blank slates". The skills required of a therapist are considered teachable, and are not contingent on the therapist's pre-existing or innate attributes, such as temperament or personality. The alternate perspective purports that trainee therapists already possess the personality characteristics and foundational skills necessary to become a therapist. This second model follows the logic that therapists typically assumed the role of helper as a child and were identified by families as peacekeepers and facilitators. Temperament and expectations are thought to inform the decision to pursue therapy as a profession. The role of training is therefore to assist the therapist in honing skills and applying these in a professional manner (Hackney & Cormier, 2012).

Much research and writing has also considered factors that motivate individuals to enter the profession of therapy. This includes a need to heal themselves from psychological distress or to resolve trauma through helping others (Adams, 2024; Cozolino, 2004; Kottler, 2010).

Stages of therapist development

Often, trainees feel a sense of over-responsibility for patients and the outcomes of therapy. They may think themselves to be the heroes in the room, while those at later career stages view the patient to be the hero. For some trainees, this can be overwhelming and may lead to a feeling of being consumed by all things therapy and being hyper-focused on patients and their prognosis. Somewhat ironically, this obsessive thinking can lead to less-optimal therapeutic outcomes. The core characteristics and differences of each stage of training and work as a therapist are summarised in Table 1.1.

Table 1.1 Typical characteristics of each developmental stage.

	Stage 1: Trainee	Stage 2: Early-career	Stage 3: Established
Therapeutic skills	Heavy use of textbooks and rules. Acquisition of technical skills. Rigidity in therapeutic thinking. Compartmentalised approach to therapy and skills.	Increased integration of skills. Greater exploration of novel skills. Comfortable in implementing new skills and approaches.	Sophisticated integration of skills and knowledge.
Therapeutic modality	Focused on mastering one therapeutic modality. Informed by training institute or supervisors/ teachers.	Increased breadth and knowledge of several therapeutic modalities/ interventions. May become aligned with a specific therapeutic modality/ intervention and seek training in a specific therapeutic modality/ intervention.	Confident in a range of therapeutic modalities and interventions. Likely to specialise in a specific therapeutic modality.
Supervision	Typically provided by training institute or employer. Focused on skill development.	May be provided or supplemented by employer. Greater autonomy in selection of supervisor.	Focused on process issues (i.e., transference) rather than content.
Identity	Self-conscious of own presence in room. Sense of over-responsibility for patient and therapeutic outcomes.	Better able to separate self from patient and therapeutic outcomes. Begins to form identity beyond that prescribed by training course or supervisors.	Greater focus on patient. Increased ability to separate self from patient.

Stage 1: Trainee therapist

The focus of this stage of training is gathering specific knowledge and technical expertise. Learning is gradual and segmented. Trainees naturally find it challenging to consolidate the volume of knowledge and skills acquired during this time. As such, trainee therapists may feel their delivery of therapy to be clunky, as they are working towards integrating theory and practice (Cozolino, 2004). Typically, trainees are hyper-aware of their own actions and overly conscious of their presence in the therapy room.

Trainees rely heavily on rules and textbooks. They may source or create their own written "scripts" for therapy sessions. This is an attempt to control and mitigate all variables during interactions with patients. Trainees are heavily influenced by teachers and supervisors, sometimes to the point of imitation. Strong identification with specific established therapists will see trainees mirror therapeutic styles; this is usually a precipitant of becoming aligned with one specific therapeutic modality, such as CBT or ACT (Carlson, 2011).

Becoming a therapist is time-consuming and, at times, arduous (McWilliams, 1999). Trainees often experience anxiety and stress, especially around starting one-on-one, face-to-face sessions with patients. These concerns are heightened by role ambiguity and lack of clarity about scope and breadth of skills expected of trainees. Trainees often express concern about inadvertently practising beyond the scope of their competence, while also reporting worry about meeting patients' needs and being able to treat all presentations. Some feel an expectation to provide a salve for all ails. These concerns point to the challenge of striking an appropriate balance between confidence and competence.

McWilliams (1999) used dream analysis to investigate trainees' anxieties. Her observations of trainees' worries were consistent with concerns identified elsewhere in the literature: separation and loss of personal support network (due to being away from home and separated from loved ones during training), low self-esteem, lack of empathy and understanding from authority figures such as supervisors and instructors, and concerns about bureaucratic directives overriding clinical judgement.

Stage 2: Early-career therapist

Defined here as therapists in the first five to ten years of practice, early-career marks the transition from intense supervision and close guidance to the development of autonomy and individual therapeutic style. Graduates often work as interns and receive regular and formal supervision as part of their employment.

First, the good news. Research consistently shows that early-career therapists provide similarly effective therapeutic outcomes as those of later-stage therapists. Now, the less positive news. Early-career therapists are unlikely to *feel* effective, at least for a while. This reflects increased insight into their own level of knowledge and experience, rather than actual incompetence.

Early-career therapists report a sense of professional freedom, while paradoxically experiencing internal and external pressure to "professionalise" their therapeutic style and performance. They will typically explore training or specialisation in one or more specific therapeutic modalities and interventions, branching out beyond the modality about which they were provided instruction during training. This individuation from instructors and supervisors can be a time of tension for therapists.

Therapists in this career stage typically begin to let go of their own concerns and cease feeling constantly self-conscious. Thus, they become free enough to start to experience their patient's concerns (Hackney & Cormier, 2012).

Early-career therapists begin to find a personal model of therapy. In this way, they become better attuned to patients' needs and realities. They are less pre-occupied and concerned about their own place in the therapy room and instead focus on the patient. Increased insight occurs regarding transference and the contribution of their own personality and experiences to patient outcomes, having become better able to use their own life experiences (both positive and negative) to enrich and enhance their work as therapists.

Stage 3: Established therapist

Established therapists exhibit a sophisticated working style. Characteristics include positive regard for patients, high congruence of professional and personal values, capacity to repair therapeutic ruptures, and use of appropriate self-disclosure (Norcross, 2011). This refined presentation is analogous to the final construction of a patchwork quilt – many separate pieces of fabric, often created over a long period of time, come together to make a final product.

Accumulation of years of experience is only one aspect of being an established therapist. Additionally, reaching this career stage involves the refinement of cognitive and emotional attributes and ongoing development of relational abilities and interpersonal skills (Skovholt & Jennings, 2004). Established therapists operate on a learned instinctive level without relying on textbook rules (Carlson, 2011). Expertise is characterised by the move from using decontextualised theory to adopting an internalised form of psychotherapy based on experiences and reflection.

How to use this book

The aim of this book is to provide trainee and early-career therapists with a resource to support both professional and personal development. Inherent to the structure and content is the assumption that therapists are at exactly the place they should be, in terms of both thinking and learning. Just as water finds its level, therapists find their place. Therapists should resist being pressured (by internal or external forces) to rush through their career. Within this text, therapists are encouraged to take one step at a time, showing themselves (and others) patience and kindness. Being a therapist is a lifelong learning opportunity; the more that is learned, the more there is to learn.

Trainee therapists will most likely find the initial chapters of this book most helpful. Aspects covered in later chapters (business considerations, countering burnout) will likely be of emerging interest to therapists with further years of work experience.

The structure of this book is designed to reflect the typical queries of therapists during the training and early-career stages. I consider that a question or quandary being repeatedly asked by trainee and early-career therapists to be an indication of a need for further information; this represents not a failing of individual therapists, but rather a potential shortfall in specific areas of the training and education system. As I tell supervisees, there is no such thing as a stupid question. But through personal and professional experiences, I know that it may not always be easy or appropriate to pose questions. While this book is not a replacement for supervision, I hope it may provide some initial answers to questions and queries common to trainee and early-career therapists that may otherwise go unasked or unanswered.

First, there is being in the room with a client. This represents an omnipresent concern for many novice therapists, with the long-held dream of beginning clinical work often mitigated by worries related to the "how-to" of therapy: keeping to time in session, building therapeutic rapport, containing talkative clients, or, conversely, encouraging reluctant clients to engage in conversation. Factors prescient to trainee and early-career therapists are the focus of subsequent chapters. These include issues such as confidentiality, professional boundaries, ethical decision-making, and transference and countertransference. Finally, information related to business considerations and supervision are offered in the final chapters. These may be more distal concerns for trainee and early-career therapists; supervision may be a training or internship provision, and business considerations (such as entering into private practice) should be contemplated only after completion of training and establishment of core therapy skills. This scaffolding approach seeks to provide sufficient information appropriate for trainee and early-career therapists, while giving an indication of future directions and possibilities in the career of a therapist. Resources and references are provided throughout for further reading.

Call-out boxes feature "words of wisdom", contributed by therapists who were once beginners. Now at various stages of their careers and from a range of therapeutic disciplines and backgrounds, these valuable insights demonstrate the breadth of knowledge and diverse experiences acquired throughout the working life of therapists.

The case studies and examples used throughout this book include de-identified, composite, and fictional information. No person, therapist, or patient is identifiable.

A note on the terminology and phrases used throughout this book. The specific terms of *therapist* and *patient* are used to maintain consistency, acknowledging that varied terms for both therapist and patient are used across and within different professions and therapeutic modalities. "Therapist" is used in reference to any person who provides therapy. "Patient" is synonymous with client or consumer and is used here to describe the recipient of therapy.

**

I hope this book will be useful for trainee and early-career therapists. I hope it brings some levity and guidance to this field of work, which can contain both sorrow and joy, sometimes simultaneously. I hope it provides a reliable source of information for when the inevitable challenges of working as a therapist arise. I hope this book will provide an opportunity for reflection on the growth that will be experienced by all therapists, including the rewards, challenges, gains, and losses.

It is important to acknowledge the scope of this book, including its limitations:

- It is not a replacement for supervision. Supervision comes in many forms – individual, group, or self-supervision. Whichever form is engaged in (ideally, it should be a combination of all of the afore-mentioned), therapists are encouraged to relish the opportunity and capitalise on the time and knowledge afforded by the opportunity of supervision. Supervision is a space in which to learn, grow, and observe. Ideally, it will be a process during which you can be honest, express humility and vulnerability, challenge yourself, identify (and perhaps confront) your preconceptions and biases. Supervision is discussed in Chapter 10.
- This book is not a script for therapy sessions. Suggested phrases and statements are just that – suggestions. Therapists all find their own voice, style, and therapeutic groove.
- It is not theoretical or academic. The focus of this book is on the practical aspects of therapy. Therapy provision is not based on guesswork, nor guided by intuition; sound theoretical knowledge is absolutely essential to working effectively as a therapist. Every aspect of work as a therapist – session content, treatment planning, reports, decision-making – should be informed by and grounded within a thorough understanding of well-established theory.
- Professional identity is inextricably linked to a therapeutic style and will inevitably inform the way in which therapy is delivered. Identity development as a therapist is a seminal and important topic. Given this, some aspects of this book contain inferences or indications towards therapist identity and its formation. The focus of this book, however, is on the practical aspects of becoming a therapist.

The identity of helping professionals and "healers" has been an important topic for eons. Ancient Greek philosophers, such as Plato and Hippocrates, wrote about the intertwinement between spiritual and physical health, establishing early ideas about evidence-based treatment and the responsibility of physicians to provide appropriate care for patients afflicted by illness or disease. The rejection of the idea of disease being caused by the supernatural was a seminal step towards an understanding of disease as biological, shaping physicians' interaction with and treatment of patients and providing for the idea of psychological aspects of well-being (Brennan & Houde, 2022).

More recently, Carl Rogers (1961) provided a foundational understanding of therapists' development of personal and professional self. Together with Gordon Allport and Abraham Maslow, Rogers developed a new perspective in psychotherapy, taking a client-centred approach and encouraging growth and development in patients and, by extension, therapists.

Rogers's theories and writings remain relevant today. His seminal text, *On Becoming a Person*, is essential reading for all therapists and helping professionals.

Further to Rogers, Irvin Yalom's (2017) autobiography, *Becoming Myself*, provides an insightful and comprehensive recall of his long and esteemed career as a psychiatrist and psychotherapist, including the development of his interest and expertise in existential psychotherapy and group therapy. Glen Gabbard (2005) also considers therapist identity formation and development, focused on the juxtaposition of theory, personality, training, and reflective practice. Kottler (2010) and Cozolino (2004) have also authored well-known texts about therapist identity formation.

- This book is not a replacement for any professional code, such as a code of ethics or code of conduct. No book or resource is a substitution for these. Codes also change over time, and it is imperative for all therapists, regardless of level of training or years of experience, to ensure currency of knowledge regarding ethical and professional conduct.
- Therapists are bound by the laws and legislation relevant to the country and state in which they practise. This book in no way replaces legal advice and is not intended to be consulted for specific legal matters. Always seek supervision around legal, ethical, and professional issues.
- The contents of this book and the ideas contained within it are largely reflective of my professional and personal experiences. It is therefore necessarily subjective. While the content is supported by referenced material and includes evidence-based information, it primarily reflects my professional perspective.
- Like all therapists, I am still learning. And much of my learning comes not only from working with patients, but working with trainees and supervisees. To this end, I look forward to hearing readers' views and perceptions of the information presented here.

Summary

- Becoming a therapist is a demanding and arduous process. It is typified by experiences common to trainee and early-career therapists.
- Common queries and concerns include keeping to time in session, engaging reluctant patients, managing "imposter syndrome", maintaining efficient and effective strategies around note-keeping and report writing, and feeling burnt out.
- Identity development of therapists is generally sequential; however, it may not be linear for all therapists at all times. Trainee therapists

typically demonstrate insecurity and dependence in their work, while established therapists exhibit independence and creativity.

- There is no shortcut to becoming a competent therapist. Skill development takes time. Practice, reflection, observation, and supervision are all necessary components of this process.
- No book or tool can provide a "script" for being a therapist, nor for running a therapy session. Over time, therapists will naturally find their own therapeutic style and voice.
- Training pathways and registration requirements to becoming a therapist differ across and between jurisdictions. It is the responsibility of each therapist to keep current knowledge of relevant registration and licensing requirements.

Note

1   Training and registration pathways to becoming a therapist vary greatly across jurisdictions. Licensing and registration requirements also change over time. Here, I outline my own experience of study and training in Australia in the mid-2000s.

Reference list

Adams, M. (2024). *The myth of the untroubled therapist* (2nd ed.). Routledge.

Brennan, J. F., & Houde, K. A. (2022). Psychological foundations in ancient Greece. In *History and systems of psychology* (pp. 36–58). Cambridge University Press.

Carlson, J. (2011). *Becoming a psychodynamic psychotherapist* [PhD thesis, Karolinska Institute].

Clarke, V. (2010). *The psychological birth of a psychotherapist: What are the parallels, if any, between becoming a mother and becoming a psychotherapist?* [PhD thesis, Auckland University].

Cozolino, L. (2004). *The making of a therapist*. Norton.

Denny, B. (2023, November 9). Self-diagnosis is on the rise, but is TikTok really to blame? *The Age*.

Gabbard, G. O. (2005). *Psychodynamic psychiatry in clinical practice* (4th ed.). American Psychiatric Publications.

Hackney, H. L., & Cormier, S. (2012). *The professional counselor: A process guide to helping* (7th ed.). Pearson.

Kottler, J. A. (2010). *On being a therapist*. Jossey-Bass.

McWilliams, N. (1999). *Psychoanalytical case formulation*. Guilford Press.

Norcross, J. C. (2011). *Psychotherapy relationships that work: Evidence-based responsiveness.* Oxford University Press.

Reising, G. N., & Daniels, M. H. (1983). A study of Hogan's model of counselor development and supervision. *Journal of Counseling Psychology, 30*(2), 235–244. https://doi.org/10.1037/0022-0167.30.2.235

Rogers, C. R. (1961). *On becoming a person: A therapist's view of psychotherapy.* Constables.

Rønnestad, M. H., & Skovholt, T. M. (2003). The journey of the counselor and therapist: Research findings and perspectives on professional development. *Journal of Career Development, 30,* 5–44.

Skovholt, T. M., & Jennings, L. (2004). *Master therapists: Exploring expertise in therapy and counseling.* Allyn and Bacon.

Yalom, I. D. (2017). *Becoming myself: A psychiatrist's memoir.* Scribe Publications.

Being in the room

The first therapy session

2

The eminent psychotherapist Harry Stack Sullivan once defined therapy as a meeting of two people, with one person less anxious than the other (Berman, 2019). The presumption here is that patients are usually anxious about attending therapy; however, trainee and early-career therapists also feel anxious, particularly prior to conducting their first therapy session.

Commencing therapy work with patients is a long-held aspiration for many students of psychology, helping professions, and other related fields in which human behaviour is studied. Many years of study culminate to one moment – the therapist sitting in a room with a patient. This innocuous-sounding event is the source of much stress and anxiety for many novice therapists. Thinking of the eustress (positive stress or adaptive stress, as opposed to the negative stress described by *distress*) associated with this situation is one explanation for the common feeling of trepidation experienced by therapists during their first session.

The first therapy session

Before turning attention to the structure of a first session, here are some general points to keep in mind when commencing work with patients:

1. Focus on clinically relevant information.
   Collecting clinically relevant information means focusing on information related to the referral reason or presenting problem. Patients have often lived long and interesting lives. Many have intriguing stories and complicated personal lives. But an initial therapy session is not an

DOI: 10.4324/9781003533030-2

interview for the patient's autobiography; it is not possible nor necessary to gather all details on every aspect of the patient's life from birth to the current moment. Rather, think of this first therapy session as a synopsis of the patient's life. Maintain a focus on the referral reason or presenting problem.

Also note that patients are often unable or unwilling to reveal all pertinent information in the first session. This may be due to timidity, embarrassment, lack of insight, inability to discern relevant and irrelevant information, or, in some cases, secondary gain (i.e., the presenting problem has an adaptive quality and therefore the problem being resolved presents a threat at some level of their psyche) (Gabbard, 2005).

2. Keep the referral question front and centre, both in your mind and in the session.

Remind yourself of the referral reason prior to the session commencing. Write the referral reason at the top of your note pad. For example, "relationship concerns", "low mood", "social anxiety", "difficulties at work", "parenting stress".

Referring to this can help keep the initial session on track and minimise collection of superfluous information. If session content segues or becomes tangential, a clear reminder of the referral reason can assist the therapist in bringing the conversation back to the reason the patient has presented for therapy.

3. Prioritise time management and keeping to time in session.

Start as you intend to continue. Punctuality (commencing and finishing a session on time) is important to establish in the first session. It is also easier to maintain punctuality if normalised from the start of the therapeutic relationship. This communicates to patients the duration and structure of sessions, setting their expectations for future sessions. It can be difficult to rein sessions back to a standard therapeutic hour (50 minutes) when the duration of previous sessions has been variable or reactive.

Remember, all information need not be collected in this first session. Cover the essentials; therapists should remind themselves (and their patients) that extra information can be discussed in future sessions.

Some therapists conduct longer intake sessions (usually 90 minutes); clearly communicating this session duration to patients helps set expectations about the duration of subsequent sessions.

4. Focus on the patient.

Many trainee and early-career therapists are understandably nervous about commencing therapy work with patients. Feeling self-conscious can lead to the therapist focusing on themselves, rather than the patient.

Avoiding the use of "I" statements is one relatively straightforward way to ensure focus remains on the patient. Commencing a statement or sentence with "I" can inadvertently put attention on the therapist and their experience of the session, rather than the patient and their needs. At times, "I" statements are appropriate, but should be used sparingly and reserved for statements that require emphasis or in which it is appropriate for the therapist to directly express their professional opinion.

For instance, "I would like to ask some questions about your sleep" can be rephrased to "how has your sleep been?". "I want to give you some information about our clinic" can be rephrased to "here is some information about our clinic". "I am happy with the treatment goals we have set" can be rephrased to "the treatment goals seem appropriate". These small changes to sentence structure and phrasing can be useful in removing focus from the therapist, thus promoting a collaborative therapeutic relationship.

Practising these statements outside of session makes for an easier and more natural integration in session. Practise this in your everyday conversations with family and friends; it can be challenging at first, but like any skill, it will soon become a habit rather than an exception.

5. Be authoritative, not authoritarian.
These phonetically similar words are sometimes erroneously used interchangeably. However, the approach encouraged by each differs in important ways.

Authoritarian suggests the therapist to be a figure who should be obeyed and whose advice is to be heeded. Conversely, authoritative suggests the therapist to be knowledgeable and trustworthy. Information is delivered with confidence, but without force.

Trainee and early-career therapists often fall into advice-giving or approval-giving mode. The style mimics an instructor or a teacher, rather than a therapist. This may be a consequence of feeling anxious, or an indication of a subconscious need to assert expertise. Therapists who have previously worked in other fields such as teaching or tutoring may also naturally fall into this type of interaction.

The alternative to this – an authoritative approach – is consistent with therapy being a joint endeavour between therapist and patient. An authoritative style encourages a collaborative therapy in which concerns can be shared and understood. This also acknowledges the power differential that exists in therapeutic relationships – the therapist has knowledge and skill which puts them in a position in which they are able to assist the patient.

> *"When you start out, you might be filled with a sense you have a great deal of knowledge to impart to others. Resist this temptation."*

Preparing for the first session

The work of the initial session begins long before the first meeting of therapist and patient. Depending on the therapist's work setting, this may include an intake phone conversation, triage (to consider urgency and ensure appropriateness of referral), and collecting information or documents such as referral paperwork.

Initial patient contact and preparation for the first therapy session will be guided by the organisation or setting in which the therapist is working. Training organisations typically provide clear structure and procedures related to intake and registration of new patients.

In many settings, intake and triage will be completed by administrative personnel. In some training organisations, students or trainee therapists conduct intake as a compulsory part of their internship or coursework. This contributes to learning and is often counted towards training hours. Intake is usually conducted via a telephone interview. This is an opportunity to gather essential referral information, including the patient's demographic or contact details, and information related to the presenting problem. Information regarding fees and informed consent can be provided to the patient. Where relevant, informed consent should also include information related to the structure and process of training clinics, specifically noting the role of trainee therapists in working under the supervision and guidance of experienced therapists.

Intake also provides an opportunity for referral triage. In this context, triage refers to ascertaining the appropriateness of the referral and evaluating its urgency. The patient's presenting problem may not be suitable for the therapist or the setting in which they work. Training clinics typically screen for referrals where the patient's concerns are related to drug and alcohol use, court-mandated therapy, patients who are in crisis or present with a high level of risk of harm to self or others, forensic patients, or those seeking specific assessment or diagnosis for funding purposes. In instances of uncertainty around the appropriateness of a referral, the patient information should be presented to a senior therapist or duty supervisor before an initial appointment is scheduled.

An initial appointment should be confirmed in writing, such as via email. Appointment reminders may also be sent via email or text message. Useful supplementary information may include directions to the clinic and information about car parking, instructions for joining a video or telephone session (for telehealth sessions), paperwork related to informed consent, and information about fees and payment, including costs related to non-attendance or late cancellation.

Conducting the first session

Here, a template is offered for an initial patient session. It is tailored for an adult therapy patient; however, it is applicable for initial sessions with other patient populations such as children (in which case the parent of caregiver usually attends without the child) or adolescents.

Note that training institutions and organisations often provide templates or checklists for initial sessions, based on specific presentations or client populations. The template in Figure 2.1 can be used in conjunction with these. Typically, therapists will draw upon several templates or guides, eventually amalgamating these to form their own structure.

Compartmentalising the initial session into clear sections represents a useful way to manage time and content. This is illustrated in Figure 2.1. The model allows for a standard 50-minute intake session but can be modified for therapists who opt for longer initial sessions, such as a 90-minute duration. Each section is detailed next.

Informed consent

It is essential to gain informed consent before commencing therapy. Informed consent relates to the patient's understanding of the risks, benefits, and alternatives to therapy. This information is necessary for a patient to make a reasoned decision about engaging in treatment.

The patient must be deemed competent to make a decision around informed consent. It is the responsibility of the therapist to ascertain competence, in relation to age, cognitive capacity, and absence of undue influence.

Therapists working with families and children must also be mindful of special considerations related to informed consent. This includes being cognisant of legislation and regulations related to obtaining informed consent from minors and when providing therapy to families and children

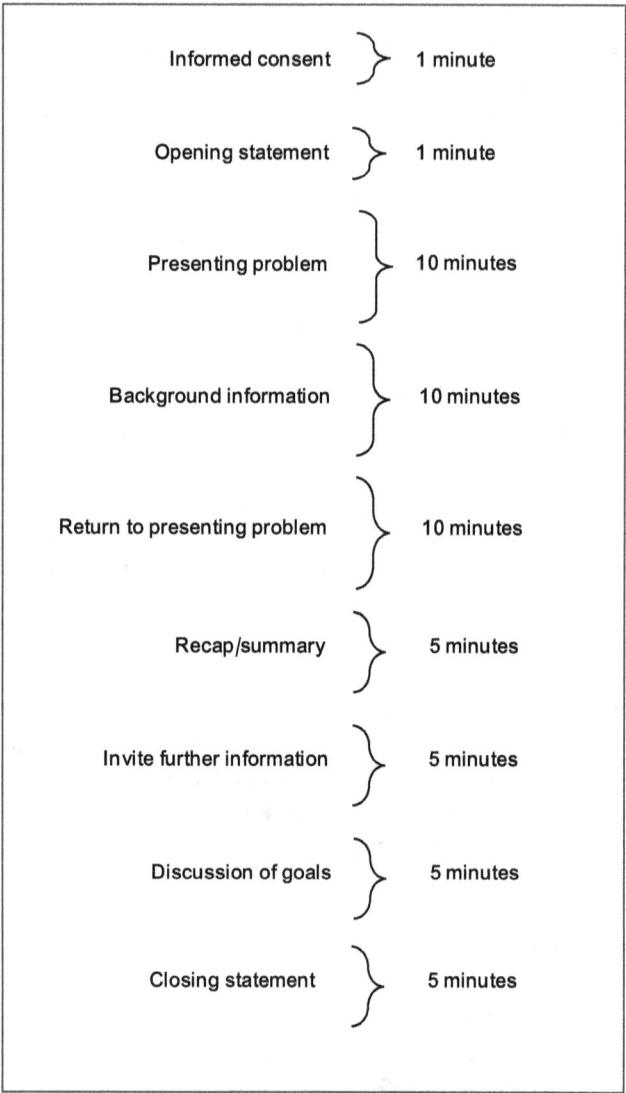

Figure 2.1 First session template.

where divorce, separation, or other legal proceedings related to custody may be relevant. Typically, up until the age of 14 years, children have informed consent provided by their parent or legal caregiver. However, this differs across jurisdictions, and legislation changes over time; it is the responsibility of each therapist to be aware of the regulations and processes applicable to their practice and patients. Younger children can still participate in the informed consent process by providing assent to treatment (Barnett et al., 2014). During this process, the child is provided with information in age-appropriate language and terminology. The aim of this is to aid the child's understanding of therapy and the process that their caregivers or parents have given permission for the young person to engage in.

Written information related to informed consent is typically presented in a short document of one to three pages in length. A copy of the document should be provided to the patient prior to engaging in therapy. A signed copy is to be kept on the patient's file. Informed consent is most often completed via an electronic or online form, but it may also be completed in paper format.

Therapists must familiarise themselves with details of informed consent relevant to the specific jurisdiction and field in which they work. Relevant aspects will depend on the setting in which the therapist works and the patient population with whom the therapist works, but will likely include:

- Confidentiality and limits to confidentiality (see Chapter 4).
- Secure storage of notes and records (see Chapter 7).
- Fee schedule and billing information, including cancellation policy (see Chapter 11).
- Contingency information in case of the therapist's unexpected incapacitation or death (see Chapter 11).

During the initial session, a brief verbal statement about informed consent is usually sufficient. There is generally no need to repeat information or give extra material beyond that which has been reviewed and signed by the patient prior to attending the initial therapy session. Some patients may also be familiar with the process of informed consent from previous engagement in therapy. Patients who, for whatever reason, have not completed an intake form prior to presenting to the first session should be encouraged to do so before the therapy session commences. Be mindful here of the reason the patient has not completed the form; they may need assistance in instances of concerns regarding literary or language barriers.

The reiteration of informed consent at the beginning of a first session may be phrased in the following way:

> Thank you for completing and signing the paperwork. To reiterate important aspects of informed consent, everything we discuss is held

confidential. There are some limits to confidentiality: first, if you or someone else is at risk of harm; second, if I am subpoenaed by a court of law to share information; and third, if you give me permission to share information with another person, such as your referring doctor.

Trainee or early-career therapists may also add that information collected in session will be shared with clinical supervisors as part of the therapist's training or supervision programme.

Typically, patients are eager to start discussing the concern that has brought them to therapy. Information about informed consent can be kept brief while conveying its importance. Just like therapy itself, informed consent is not "one size fits all"; patients who, for reasons such as cognitive impairment, language, or cultural considerations, will likely require a more thorough reiteration of informed consent. The therapist is required to use clinical judgement in these situations; if a patient seems confused or inattentive to an explanation of informed consent, the therapist should clarify the patient's understanding and provide further information as needed.

Informed consent is a dynamic rather than static process. As therapy progresses and new information is shared, the therapist should revisit and explain relevant aspects of informed consent in order to ensure the patient's ongoing understanding around confidentiality. The therapist can flag this by inviting the patient to ask any questions related to informed consent:

> Let me know if you have any further queries about informed consent, either now or at a later time. We can revisit the information at any time.

Opening statement

Patients attending an initial therapy session are usually eager to "tell their story". For many, this may be the first opportunity to speak about the concern or problem that has led them to engage with a therapist. Most patients are therefore understandably eager to talk and need little coaxing to share information. The patient will likely appreciate the therapist avoiding distractions such as excessive small talk. There is no need to "fill the space" or "fill the time"; this is the patient's time to tell their story. Allowing the patient to speak freely for the first part of the therapy session usually pre-emptively provides answers to many of the questions that the therapist may be planning to pose.

Some therapists, particularly those from a psychodynamic or psychoanalytic modality, may not use an opening statement. Instead, silence is used. Saying nothing and providing no prompt invites the patient to initiate the conversation.

Most therapists, however, provide a brief opening statement or question. Some ideas may be:

"Tell me, what brings you in today?"
"What ails you?" (Yalom, 2009)
"Where shall we begin?" (Perel, 2006)
"Can you tell me about the reason you sought the referral?"
"Today is about hearing from you, about what has been happening in your world."

Some patients may say they "don't know where to start". Dependent on the patient and their presentation, the therapist offering an encouraging statement or prompt may be useful:

"Start wherever feels right. We will make sense of the information together."
"Would you like me to ask you some questions to get us started?"

Information about presenting problem

Listen to the patient. Allow the patient time and space to speak uninterrupted, for about ten minutes.

It is likely that the therapist will need to say very little during this time. Typically, patients will give much of the necessary information about their concerns without the need for a specific list of questions. The patient is the expert on their own life and the happenings within it. There is usually little need to ask patients specific questions during this brief time; the idea here is to allow patients to freely express themselves and initiate the patient to the idea of being able to talk freely about their concerns within a therapy session. Here, the therapist can keep in mind the queries and points requiring clarification, holding them over for later in the session.

During this time, microskills (nodding, facial expressions) and brief reflective statements can be used to indicate the therapist's interest and understanding of the patient's concerns.

After about ten minutes, the therapist can introduce a summary statement. This provides a brief synopsis of the information presented thus far by the patient. For example, for a patient referred for concerns related to low mood, a statement such as the following may be appropriate:

> Thank you for sharing your thoughts. From what you've said so far, it seems that over the past couple of months you've been feeling really flat. At times you've been especially emotional and teary, which is not usual for you. And you've not had the usual motivation to do the things you enjoy, like going out with your friends or attending football games.

The following example is for a patient referred following a motor vehicle accident, with symptoms consistent with post-traumatic stress disorder.

> Since the car accident about eight months ago, it seems you've felt really down. Others have commented on this change in your mood. And, as you put it, you've been "jumping at shadows". You've also had trouble sleeping, with nightmares some evenings, too. Since the car accident you've been able to drive again, but the thought of being a passenger in a car brings on distressing thoughts and intense anxiety.

A further example is for a patient ambivalent about attending therapy, who may be less forthcoming with initial information:

> Your parents encouraged you to come along today. It seems they've been worried about the amount of time you've been spending online, particularly with gaming. You've said you're not so concerned about this. But you did mention feeling a bit out of sorts, especially since leaving school last year?

The therapist should check in with the patient for accuracy of information. For example:

> "Have I got that right?"
> "Does that reflect your experience?"
> "Am I missing anything important, so far?"
> "Just checking that we're both on the same page here . . ."

Broader background information

The focus of the initial session is on the referral reason or presenting problem. Collecting general background information is also important, as this helps understand the broader aspects of the patient's life and the context in which the presenting problem exists.

This can be introduced by a brief statement, such as:

"Now, let's zoom out a little, to get an understanding of other aspects of your life."
"I'm interested to hear more about your life . . ."

Sufficient background information can be gathered in around ten minutes. Remember, this is an initial therapy session, not a detailed account of the patient's entire life. The focus should be on aspects of the patient's life relevant to the presenting problem. This helps contain both the therapist and patient and will assist in keeping the session to time.

This part of the initial session benefits from the use of open-ended questions. In comparison to closed questions, open-ended questions offer an efficient way of gathering richer information. For example, "Do you live at home?" may elicit a dichotomous response (yes/no) that will require further probing, but a query such as "Who lives at home?" invites the patient to share further information.

Also be mindful here of asking questions that reflect the therapist's own interests rather than being open to the patient's unique experiences. For example, asking a patient when they last saw a movie at the cinema or the title of the last book they read might reflect the therapist's interest but not be consistent with the patient's interests; a patient's participation (or lack thereof) tells us little about the patient's behaviour. At best, it indicates scant information, while at worst it may alienate the patient by making them feel "othered" and judged by a therapist who seems to expect the patient to share interests similar to their own. Open-ended questions such as "What do you do for fun?", followed up with "When was the last time you did that?", gives information relevant to the patient, and demonstrates the therapist's attention and care towards them.

Some useful open-ended questions are listed in Table 2.1.

At the end of this time, the therapist should offer a brief summary of the information shared by the patient. This can then lead to a return to the presenting problem.

Table 2.1 Open-ended questions to gain information about patient's lives.

Question	Purpose
"Who lives at home?"	To ascertain family composition and family dynamics. This open-ended question does not assume all patients' families to be nuclear, not are assumptions made about typical composition of a household or home.
"How does everyone in your family get along?"	To ascertain general family dynamics.
"What do you do for fun?"	To gain an idea of the patient's social life and interests.
"What are your hobbies?"	To learn about the patient's usual leisure activities and areas of interest. To build rapport.
"When was the last time you did that activity?"	To gain an indication of anhedonia (loss of interest in pleasurable activities).
"Who do you spend time with, outside of work?"	To gauge social support and the social context in which the patient lives.
"How is your sleep?" "What changes have you noticed in your appetite?"	To gain information about symptoms that may indicate depression, anxiety, or order areas of distress.
"Talk me through a typical day for you."	To gain an indication of the patient's typical daily activities.

For example,

> Thanks for that extra information. Just to summarise – and let me know if I'm getting this right – you live with your wife and two kids. Your wife's parents are often around to help with the kids, and your folks live a few hours' drive away.
>
> Work feels stable at the moment, but you've been a bit worried about ongoing redundancies within the company. You used to really enjoy playing and watching sport, but this has dropped off since the birth of your second child around three years ago. Between work and family, it seems hard to find time for the things you enjoy?

Return to presenting problem

Then, return to the presenting problem. This can be done by overtly sig-
nalling that the discussion will again focus on the presenting problem. For
example:

> "Let's turn our attention back to [presenting problem]."
> "Let's return to what we were talking about earlier. You were telling
> me about [presenting problem]."

Otherwise, it can be useful to link information about the patient's life to the
presenting problem. For example, for a patient who has been referred for
insomnia:

> You mentioned feeling really stressed about your studies, and that
> you've spending many hours on assignments and often work on
> these late at night. Have you experienced sleep problems at other
> times?

Here is a further example, this time for a patient referred for social
anxiety:

> It seems that you have a close group of friends. You enjoy spending
> time with this small group. But the idea of attending a party or event
> with people you don't know very well seems daunting. Can you tell
> me a little more about that?

Questions asked by the therapist will depend on the presenting problem
and the initial information garnered earlier in the session. Table 2.2
includes suggested phrasing of questions relevant to include in the first
session.

Invitation to share

It is not possible nor necessary to collect exhaustive information about a
person's life in one session, whether that session be 50 minutes, 90 minutes,
or longer. Rather, the therapist should focus on collecting pertinent information and encouraging the patient to focus on sharing pertinent information. An important component of this is to check in with the patient about

Table 2.2 Phrasing of questions useful for the first session.

Query	Sample phrases/questions
Impact of presenting problem	"What effect has this had on your life?" "If this problem continues, what ongoing impact do you think it may have on your life?"
History of concern, pattern of problem over time	"How long has this been a concern?" "Have you experienced this before?" "Is this the first time you've felt like this?" "Are there other times when this has been a problem for you?"
Attempts to manage/resolve	"What kind of things have you done to try to manage this?" "What have you found to be most helpful?" "What have you found to be most unhelpful?" "Have some things helped for a little while, but not been a permanent solution?"
Social support	"Have you talked to any of your friends or family about this?"
Perception of problem within social group	"What do your friends or family make of this?" "Have any of your friends experienced similar concerns?"
Previous therapy or help-seeking behaviour	"Have you talked to any other health professionals, such as your family doctor, about this?" "Have you seen a therapist or other mental health professional about this?" "Have you found any further information online or in books about this problem?"
Motivation for change, hope for future	"How would your life be different if we were able to get on top of [presenting problem]?" "What might life look like if we were able to make a change to this concern?" "On a scale of 1–10, how much would you like this part of your life to be different?" "How hopeful are you that this part of your life could be different?"
Risk assessment	"People sometimes have thoughts of hurting themselves or taking their own life. Is this something you have experienced?" "Sometimes people have thoughts about hurting other people. Is this something you have experienced?"

what has been shared so far, and if there are any pressing points that have not yet been discussed. For example:

> Is there anything that you would like to let me today? Anything we've not yet had a chance to talk about?
>
> We've covered a lot of ground so far. Before we move on to thinking about our work together and what our goals may look like, can I ask if there's anything you would like to mention that we haven't yet covered?
>
> You've provided a great overview of your life and what's happening for you at the moment. It's helped with my understanding of you and your life. But before we finish today, can I ask, and keeping in mind that we can continue talking about this in our next session – is there anything you would like to mention that we've not yet had a chance to discuss?

Goals of therapy

Gaining an understanding of the patient's purpose for presenting to therapy is an essential task of the initial session (Minuchin, 2003). This, together with building rapport and beginning to establish a therapeutic relationship, is a key factor that distinguishes a therapy session from a social conversation with a friend, family member, or other acquaintance.

Goals of therapy have usually been implied throughout the first session. These will typically flow from the information about the presenting problem and the broader information about the patient's life. Rarely will the stipulated goals come as a surprise to the therapist. A disconnect between the information presented in the initial session and the goals of treatment warrants further exploration by the therapist. This incongruence might be indicative of the first session lacking appropriate focus on the referral reason, a lack of insight on the patient's behalf, or the therapist dominating the first session to the detriment of the patient having time and space to express their thoughts or share their experiences.

Often, patients will have a fair idea about what they would like to achieve from therapy. This may be especially true of patients who have previously engaged in therapy, or those who present as psychologically literate or psychologically minded. Still, patients will most likely require assistance to articulate or elucidate goals. This makes sense, given that a patient would be unlikely to engage in therapy if they were able to clearly conceptualise and enact their own treatment goals. It is therefore the role of the therapist is to guide and inform the patient about therapy and its possible outcomes, especially at this early stage of engagement.

Therapists can provide examples to prompt the patient's thinking around this, while being cautious about ensuring this process is collaborative rather than dictated by the therapist. Suggestions around general areas common to goal-setting may be useful in encouraging the patient to think about specific goals:

- Improving mood and well-being
- Engaging in specific tasks, such as aeroplane travel
- Coping with specific events
- Improving interpersonal relationships
- Managing and/or reducing anxiety
- Decision-making about a specific problem or situation

Some patients are able to set clear and purposeful goals at the end of the first session. This is particularly true for patients who have previously engaged with therapy. For example:

> "I want to be able to take a flight on an aeroplane to take a vacation with my family this summer."
> "I want to better understand myself."
> "I want to feel happier."
> "I want to feel less anxious at social events, such as parties."
> "I want to sleep better, I want to resolve this insomnia."
> "I want to learn how to better communicate with my partner."
> "I want to worry less about work."
> "I want to make a decision about whether or not to have children."
> "I want to better understand my relationships."

Some patients may not be ready to set goals in the first session. This is especially likely if they are presenting for therapy in the context of experiencing acute distress or immediately after a traumatic event, such as soon after a motor vehicle accident, death of a loved one, or in the midst of a life transition such as the breakdown of a relationship. At this time, the patient may not have the cognitive capacity or executive function necessary to generate goals, as their mind is taxed by recalling and processing details of the stressor or situation. Goal-setting should therefore be held over to a later session.

In some instances, it may be appropriate to suggest goal-setting as a homework task. For patients who are unable to articulate goals or are ambivalent about doing so, it can be useful to "plant the seed" of goal setting. This can be done by promoting language around goal-directed treatment and encouraging consideration of treatment outcomes. For example:

> Between now and the next time we meet, try to think about how you would like to continue with the things we have talked about today. Think about what we might work towards in our sessions. For example, in talking about your problems at work with your co-worker, John, we could consider a goal about how to manage those difficulties within your workplace.

Closing statement

Indicate to the patient that the session is coming to a close. Patients need to know that the session is coming to an end, or has ended. Neither the therapist nor the patient should be surprised by an abrupt end to a therapy session.

A good way to bookend the session is to check in with the patient about their experience of the session. A "here-and-now" question about their current thoughts and feelings brings the patient back to the present moment (Yalom, 2009). This also provides an opportunity to normalise that therapy sessions – especially initial ones – can be fatiguing.

A closing statement indicates to the patient that the focus of the session is turning towards a summary or concluding moment, marking a pivot away from discussion of the referral reason or presenting problem.

This also provides an opportunity to mark the end of the session, indicating to the patient that the session time is coming to an end. For example:

> In the last couple of minutes of today's session, can I check in with you about how this hour or so has been for you?

The therapist should give the patient an indication of their thoughts the suitability of ongoing sessions.

> Given what we've talked about today, and dependent on your thoughts about continuing sessions, I believe we can work together.

Trainee or early-career therapists may need to check with a supervisor or senior therapist about the appropriateness of the referral and the capacity for ongoing work, as this may be dependent on new information garnered in the initial session. In this case, therapists should remind the patient about their training status and the supervisory relationship. For example:

> As we talked about earlier, I am working under the supervision of a senior therapist. We often discuss aspects of patient care. I'll check in with my supervisor with what we've talked about today. We can then chat further how to proceed with sessions.

Instilling hope is an important aspect of this initial session. Some therapists are overt and open with patients about their ideas of the prognosis for the patient and the viability of working together. Confidence and competence in making judgements about this comes with time; trainee and early-career therapists should maintain caution in using such explicit statements.

Statements to convey a prognosis or capacity to work together may include:

> "I think we can work together."
> "I'm hopeful that we can work together to get on top of this concern."

Resist grand statements about what can be achieved through therapy. These may please the patient (and therapist) in the moment and placate worry or anxiety about the presenting problem, but ultimately, such statements put undue pressure on the therapeutic process and its outcomes. The therapist never makes promises about their capacity to "cure" the patient or completely absolve their concerns, nor should they provide any explicit guarantee about the effectiveness of intervention or treatment. This is both unethical and unprofessional.

Instead, the therapist can talk in general terms about the process and efficacy of specific treatments, noting individual differences and tailoring the information in a way that the patient can comprehend. Providing a balance between being realistic and being hopeful is a useful approach for both therapist and patient. The therapist should also check in with the patient about their understanding of the treatment, its potential benefits and consequences, and alternatives to the treatment being discussed (including the impact of not receiving any treatment). This is in keeping with informed consent being an ongoing and dynamic process; rather than a statement or agreement made at the start of therapy, informed consent is revisited as new information, such as treatment, is discussed.

If appropriate, therapists can indicate the amount and frequency of sessions they anticipate working with the patient for. However, it may be more likely that this conversation will be held over until after the second or third session, when further information has been collected and the presenting problem and treatment options have been further discussed and qualified.

Summary

- Conducting an initial therapy session is often the culmination of many years of study and theoretical knowledge. This signals a rewarding but inherently challenging new stage.
- Novice therapists often report feelings of trepidation or nervousness about conducting their first therapy session. This is a completely normal and legitimate reaction to a watershed moment.
- Important aspects of the first session include: collecting clinically relevant information, focusing on the presenting problem or referral reason, managing time, and building rapport with the patient.
- The initial session represents the start of a therapeutic relationship. This is an opportunity to build rapport, establish the tone and style of therapy, and provide an indication of the direction of treatment.
- Following a clear structure for the first session is beneficial for both therapist and patient. This allows relevant and necessary information to be collected in a timely and professional manner.
- The structure of the initial session facilitates exploration of the presenting problem, gathering of background information, and setting of treatment goals.
- Treatment goals are an essential part of therapy. Integral here is striking a balance between instilling hope for the patient while ensure a realistic perspective on achievable and realistic therapeutic outcomes.

Reference list

Barnett, J. E., Zimmerman, J., & Walfish, S. (2014). *The ethics of private practice: A practical guide for mental health clinicians*. Oxford University Press.

Berman, J. (2019). *Writing the talking cure: Irvin D. Yalom and the literature of psychotherapy*. State University of New York.

Gabbard, G. O. (2005). *Psychodynamic psychiatry in clinical practice* (4th ed.). American Psychiatric Publications.

Minuchin, S. (2003). *Families & family therapy* (29th ed.). Harvard University Press.

Perel, E. (2006). *Mating in captivity: Unlocking erotic intelligence*. Harper.

Yalom, I. D. (2009). *The gift of therapy: Reflections on being a therapist*. Harper Perennial.

Staying in the room

3

Beyond the first session

Subsequent therapy sessions provide an opportunity for the therapist and patient to build upon the foundations established in the initial session. This includes continuing to build rapport, collecting further information about the referral reason or presenting problem, and learning more about the patient's broader life and the context in which the presenting problem is being experienced.

Therapy sessions vary greatly in terms of content and format. There is no one set formula, nor is there a right or wrong way of conducting a session. Content, style, and approach are dependent upon various factors, such as patient presentation and symptomatology, therapeutic modality, and anticipated length of treatment or number of sessions. Whatever the delivery, therapists should ensure their approach to the provision of therapy is consistent, evidence-based, informed by the patient and their presenting problem, and within the scope of their training and level of competence.

Trainee and early-career therapists often seek to rely on a "script" for sessions. To an extent, this is offered by manualised treatments (such as a ten-session intervention for high-prevalence conditions such as anxiety, insomnia, or social phobia). Phrases and prompts for therapists are often included in treatment manuals, together with specific content to be covered in each session. However, even the most detailed manualised treatment requires some agency and input from the therapist, in terms of verbal content and responding to patients. Attempting to provide therapy using another therapist's words will likely seem inauthentic; this insincerity impacts rapport and is detrimental to the establishment and maintenance of a therapeutic relationship.

DOI: 10.4324/9781003533030-3

Good therapy remains a dialogue, even when prescribed through means such as a treatment manual. Each therapist will necessarily develop their own style that is appropriate and reflective of their own personality, temperament, principles, training, and professional context (McWilliams, 1999). It is vitally important for a therapist to find their own voice; inspiration can be drawn from others, but the essential key ingredients to this are time and practice.

In the absence of a therapy session script being available, many novice therapists seek to create a detailed plan for dialogue, often right down to the exact words and phrases to be used. This is quite an undertaking in terms of time and effort, especially considering the many possibilities for the dialogue between patient and therapist. But the main problem is that scripting a session rarely works – patients' responses are often unpredictable, leaving a scripted therapist searching for a spontaneous response.

While we can acknowledge the task of "scripting sessions" as unhelpful and, in most cases, impossible, the desire of a novice therapist for such detailed preparation is understandable – in our academic and professional lives we are told to prepare and plan, whether for a presentation, assignment, or speech at an event. But therapy is distinct from these activities; it is a conversation between two people, rather than the delivery of a monologue. Therapy sessions are dynamic rather than static. Dialogue needs to be responsive and flexible, not scripted. However, a framework or plan *is* necessary to orient the therapist and provide therapy that is structured, evidence-based, and efficacious. Therapists can and should prepare for therapy sessions, but they cannot be wholly scripted.

"Most therapists can follow the ingredients of evidence-based, manualised treatment. The effective therapist is able to work through the curve balls."

Attempting to employ scripted conversation often results in a stilted and non-engaging therapy session. The patient may not provide the response anticipated by the therapist. This can leave both therapist and patient feeling lost – the therapist stumbles over their words, and the patient may feel they have said or done something displeasing to the therapist by not providing the "correct" response. It is akin to new parents who feel frustrated when their infant does not follow a carefully planned sleep schedule; babies don't read baby books, and therapy patients don't read treatment manuals.

Instead, trainee and early-career therapists benefit most from learning and applying core therapy skills that do not necessitate scripting. Planning is essential to therapy, but so too are flexibility and spontaneity. Striking a balance between these represents an essential clinical skill. This presents a challenging dichotomy for trainee and early-career therapists – be prepared for the expected, but also be prepared for the unexpected.

To this end, the information presented in this chapter is broad in nature. This allows the application of the information and strategies to a wide variety of therapeutic modalities, presenting problems, and patient populations. The concepts discussed here have relevance to therapists working across different contexts, with varied patient populations, and with a broad array of therapeutic modalities.

Key consideration is given to in-session skills including time management, core therapy skills such as listening and the use of silence, and rapport building and working with difficult patients. Other tasks considered include treatment planning and formulation, and terminating a therapeutic relationship. Broader occupational queries are also explored, including choosing a therapeutic modality and considerations around learning and applying diagnostic skills.

Time management

Keeping to time in session is a frequent concern for trainee and early-career therapists. Initially, some trainees and early-career therapists fear that they be unable to "fill" a whole therapeutic hour with a patient. However, most quickly realise that there is typically no shortage of content to discuss in a therapy session; finishing a session on time is a more realistic concern. Time management is a common concern for novice therapists; however, it also continues to impact the work of more experienced therapists.

A "therapeutic hour" is typically 50 minutes. This allows the scheduling of back-to-back sessions commencing on the hour, with a short break for the therapist between patients. Some therapists offer shorter or longer appointments, such as 30 or 60 minutes per session. Whichever is chosen, the importance lies in consistency; this provides structure for both therapist and patient and allows for appropriate planning of both overall treatment and individual sessions.

"We're not general practitioners or family doctors. We have 50 minutes to manage the time, and barring a complete disaster, we should be able to run on time."

Therapeutic modality and orientation strongly influence individual therapists' attitudes towards time and its management. For instance, cognitive behaviour therapy (CBT) typically adopts a strong, time-limited structure. Characteristic of CBT is a clear agenda for each session and adherence to time. Cognitive behavioural therapists are typically strict about duration of sessions and the structure and content within each session (Beck & Beck, 1995). Psychodynamic psychotherapists and psychoanalytic psychotherapists also typically adhere to strict rules around time (Gabbard, 2005).

Considering therapeutic modality and the viewing of time management through a therapeutic frame offers structure and direction for therapists. Most importantly, adhering to session time provides a consistent structure for patients; they know what to expect from sessions in terms of time, and they can plan their own time around this. Adhering to a set time in sessions is also containing for patients, sending a consistent message that their problems or concerns are manageable and treatable (Denny, 2024). Allowing session time to be dictated by the severity or complexity of the patient's concerns may communicate the message that their problems are insurmountable; the notion that a trained therapist cannot manage the patient's concerns in the allocated amount of time can precipitate or perpetuate a feeling of hopelessness or helplessness. In keeping to time, therapists can send a clear and supportive message to patients: the patients' concerns have been acknowledged and can be managed. The support around these concerns can be provided in a manner that is empathic, but that remains clear and structured. This containment can be of profound benefit for patients, particularly those with complex personality features, or those who have experienced disorganisation or chaos in their personal lives or within their family backgrounds. Containment and clarity have likely not been expressed or experienced with the patients' circle of family, friends, or social network. A framework that encompasses confidence and competence can, in and of itself, comprise the basis of a meaningful therapeutic outcome (McWilliams, 1999; Yalom, 1989; Young et al., 2007).

> *"It took years to feel comfortable*
> *with ending sessions on time, and to get how time*
> *behaves with different patients."*

From a business and financial perspective, time management and adhering to time in session is paramount. Running over time in sessions has financial implications, as extra session time represents work for which the therapist is not being directly remunerated. It is essentially unpaid work.

This can add up to a significant amount and impact the financial viability of a therapy business or organisation. Further, keeping to time in session helps avoid the domino effect of each appointment of the day running progressively late.

★★

Therapists often attribute difficulties with time-keeping to the patient. Therapists must remember, however, that patients are not expected to know "how to do" therapy. Many may be new to the process of therapy, and even those who have participated before may be now engaging in a different therapeutic modality in which structure and expectations vary.

Car owners are not expected to service their own vehicle at the mechanics. Diners at a restaurant are not asked to cook their own meal. Customers at a clothing store are not required to sew their own outfits. Analogous to these situations, patients should not be expected to have the knowledge or capacity to "do therapy" to themselves. Patients present to therapy because, for many varied reasons and usually not without concerted efforts to do so, they have been unable to resolve the problem or difficulty with which they present. To this end, therapists should be mindful of their responsibility in leading the patient through therapy sessions and course of therapy, including its structure and time management.

Common examples in which time management concerns are attributed to patients include:

- A "49er", wherein the patient raises a new issue or concern at the literal final minute of a 50-minute therapy session.
- A "door handle confession", where the patient raises a new issue or significant concern as they are leaving the consulting room.
- The patient being difficult to contain, due to being talkative, tangential, or providing overly detailed information.
- The patient providing information superfluous to the referral reason or presenting problem.
- The patient's problems being very complex and therefore requiring extra time.
- Fears of the leaving the patient "high and dry". The therapist feels unable to conclude a session when the issues or topics discussed have not been fully explored or adequately resolved.
- Situations in which the patient is in a heightened state of distress at the end of the session. The therapist therefore feels unable to finish the session on time.

To reiterate, it is the responsibility of the therapist to keep time in session. It is never the responsibility of the patient. Attribution of blame to the patient for concerns related to time-keeping is erroneous and unhelpful.

While time-keeping always remains the core responsibility of the therapist, in reality this often becomes a collaborative task, shared between therapist and patient. As the course of therapy progresses, patients often get into the flow of the 50-minute therapeutic hour and will (consciously or unconsciously) present information and content that can be considered within the session, in terms of both type and amount. Indeed, collaboration around time-keeping is one of the hallmarks of CBT; the therapist models agenda setting in initial sessions, with incremental responsibility given to patients as sessions progress (Beck & Beck, 1995). This is an example of both modelling and vicarious learning; the patient is not directly instructed to adhere to time or to pay attention to it, but many quickly develop an awareness of time and join the therapist in being cognisant of keeping to time in session.

Therapists experiencing difficulties or concerns around time-keeping is generally indicative of something more complex than simple tardiness. Therapists who find themselves running overtime in session, whether consistently or with specific patients, are encouraged to reflect on the likely contribution of personal factors and process issues to problems with time-keeping. This is one aspect of a psychological phenomenon known as countertransference. This refers to a process by which the therapist's work is impacted by factors including their feelings and thoughts about the patient, the therapist's own personal history, and current events in the therapist's professional and personal life. The phenomenon of countertransference and its role in understanding therapeutic relationships and therapeutic outcomes is detailed further in Chapter 8.

---

*"I have learned not to be so harsh on myself when time goes
really slowly with one patient (testing my concentration) and
flies by with the next (testing my subtle clock-watching skills)."*

Three broad areas are useful to consider when addressing time management. First is the therapist's relationship with time outside of their professional role. Second is those individual personality factors that shape the relationship with time. Third, it is important to consider how the therapist's management of time may reflect the patient's presentation. This last point is made with the caveat that time-keeping remains the responsibility of the therapist; however, it is acknowledged that it can be influenced by the patient.

The therapist's relationship with time outside of work can provide a good indication of their capacity for management of time during work. The therapy room is a microcosm not only for patients, but also for therapists. Here, the notion of a microcosm refers to the idea that the behaviours and mechanisms from a larger setting are apparent in a smaller setting (Yalom, 2009). Think of a petri-dish, in which scientists cultivate and observe a specimen, thus allowing generalisations to the broader environment from which the specimen was collected. A therapist's behaviour inside and outside of the therapy room will invariably share similarities; the cross-over between a therapist's professional identity and personal self is inevitable and should be explored rather than ignored or repressed (Hart, 1985). This may include running late for personal appointments or social events, or "losing track of time" while doing other tasks. Identifying the factors relevant to time management outside of work can assist in being minded about time management at work. These factors may include underestimating the time required to complete a certain task, spreading oneself too thin between tasks, agreeing to too many obligations or social invitations, neglecting to allocate a reasonable amount of time to tasks or activities, not anticipating necessary downtime or space between activities, or failing to plan ahead.

Second, consider individual and personality factors that shape the relationship with time and capacity to keep to time in the therapeutic setting. Therapists often exhibit personality features of perfectionism and unrelenting standards; this can contribute to difficulties around setting professional boundaries, including boundaries around adhering to allocated session time (Adams, 2024). Some therapists, particularly during trainee and early-career stages but sometimes extending to therapists with more years of experience, may be impacted by a "rescuer complex". That is, they feel an overwhelming need to provide care for the patient that goes beyond that expected in the role as a therapist. Giving extra time to patients in session reinforces the therapist's own identity as a "rescuer", bolstering the notion of being needed by the patient and creating a dependence or co-dependence in the therapeutic relationship. In these instances, the therapeutic relationship becomes highly subjective, rather than maintaining a healthy level of objectivity inherent and necessary to professional relationships. In extreme cases, the rescuer complex can precipitate collusion between a therapist and patient, where a lack of boundaries around time can be the beginning of a slippery slope towards lack of adherence to other parts of the professional role as therapist. This does little to progress treatment outcomes for the patient, and in some instances can be harmful (Corey et al., 2024).

"Therapists tend to be perfectionistic and self-sacrificial people who want to help and add value to their clients. This can pull them into wanting to do more and give more, and that can be really at odds with effective time management."

Last, think about how time management may be impacted by the patient and their presentation. The notion that the patient and their presentation may *contribute* to time management in session is distinct from *attributing blame* for time management difficulties to the patient. In this sense, it is imperative for the therapist to recognise and manage aspects of the patient and their presentation that may be causing challenges in keeping to time. For example, patients who present in a chaotic or disorganised manner – perhaps being tangential in jumping between several loosely related stories or unrelated topics in a short space of time – can be challenging to contain. Patients who present as chaotic or disorganised can also induce a sense of chaos or disorganisation within the therapist; this may translate to the therapist somehow mirroring or matching their behaviour, thus creating challenges around keeping to time in session.

Therapists who find themselves giving more time or energy to certain patients should also be attentive to the potential for "splitting". This psychodynamic concept refers to the tendency of some patients, particularly those with borderline or narcissistic personality features, to create a psychological rift between individual members of a group, such as a family or a treatment team. Related to therapy, this can take the form of denigrating a previous therapist (perhaps by criticising their therapeutic approach or style) while upholding the current therapist as the last vestiture of hope in absolving the patients' chronic challenges (Gabbard, 2005). For therapists, this lauding can feel good; after all, therapists are not immune to flattery, and compliments can feel especially impactful in a professional context which invariably necessitates sitting with others' difficult and often negative emotions. But therapists need to recognise this as potentially manipulative behaviour on the part of patients, whether unconscious or conscious. Rather than encouraging collaborative treatment, splitting essentially pits professionals against each other. As a general rule, a patient quick to denigrate other therapists or previous treatment teams or previous experiences may be engaging in splitting behaviour. Therapists should be aware of this, especially in instances in which extra session time is allowed in response to the notion that the current therapist is encouraged by the patient's perception of them possessing a unique style or special skill that provides unparallel promise for the patient's recovery. The role of countertransference should be considered here (see Chapter 8).

Challenges with time management can also indicate problems with planning, related to both individual sessions and overall treatment. These may require further attention, review, or modification. A comprehensive formulation is also important here; a thorough understanding of the patient and their presenting problem will help organise the therapeutic frame and the therapist's thoughts about the patient and the treatment. Coherence and clarity will inform the structure, content, and flow of sessions. Treatment planning, session planning, and formulation are all dynamic rather than static processes. Each require planning and some solidity; however, flexibility is necessary in order to allow for new information or change of opinion that may occur over time.

Feelings of overwhelm or confusion associated with the patient and their presenting problem (or problems) can also contribute to difficulties around managing time. Therapists struggling to keep to time may report that the patient's problems are simply too complex to be contained to a 50-minute session. In some ways, this seems a reasonable assumption – the more complex or numerous the problems, the harder it would seem to contain a session to a set time. Many patients present with complex or numerous problems; however, in these instances it is the role of the therapist to understand and manage the complexity, rather than get drawn into it. Here, proper case conceptualisation and formulation is imperative. Running to time sends a message of clarity and confidence – while complex, the patients' concerns and experiences are manageable. It is the role of the therapist to provide a compassionate and containing response to patients, rather than collude or join in their despair. Therapists are in the business of promoting hope, rather than encouraging hopelessness; containing patients' concerns to a set amount of time is one important way to convey optimism and confidence.

For patients with complex presentations or who report numerous concerns, it is especially helpful to revisit the patient's goals of treatment. These are usually set during initial sessions. Both therapist and patient being reminded of these agreed-upon goals of treatment can help re-centre sessions. The continued relevance and applicability of goals should also be considered, and in this instance may require reconsideration or modification. For patients whose presenting problems are numerous or complex, time management will be assisted by acknowledging this complexity and ensuring clear focus on specific goals. The selection of relevant goals should be collaborative but will also be informed by factors such as therapeutic modality and anticipated length of treatment and number of sessions. Attempting to resolve all the patient's problems will likely lead to problems with time management. Instead, setting reasonable and attainable goals for each episode of care benefits the patient and makes the therapist's work more realistic and achievable.

In summary, therapists experiencing difficulties with time management are encouraged to revisit core aspects and principles of care. This includes treatment goals, treatment planning, session plans, and formulation. These dynamic processes and the documentation related to each needs to be updated as therapy progresses, and as the therapist's understanding of the patient and their concerns evolves. A solid understanding of these will aid time management.

Time as a source of clinical information

Time can be an important source of clinical information. For example, patients arriving consistently late for sessions may represent a therapy-interfering behaviour. The tendency to raise important information in the final few minutes of a therapy session may represent avoidance, as there is no time left in the session to discuss the issue that has been belatedly raised.

Several common time management concerns are summarised in Table 3.1. Suggestions for interpretation or understanding are included, together with strategies to manage time in these instances.

Time management strategies

Some therapists have a natural tendency towards time management. Their "internal clock" is strong. They are punctual in dealings in both their personal and professional lives. They multitask with ease and seem to manage numerous demands with aplomb. These personal skills may predispose these individuals to adhering quite easily to the time-limited structure of a therapy session.

Therapists who do not have this natural tendency for time management will require purposeful attention and the application of clear and relevant strategies. Like any new skill, this requires practice and effort. Here, it is useful to remember that a new habit or skill becomes habitual after approximately six weeks of consistent application and practice.

Just like any skill, development and mastery of time management is aided by clear and relevant strategies. Strategies outlined here include: agenda setting; applying a "bell curve" rule; dividing the session in segments; and ensuring clear separation between therapy and non-therapy tasks (such as billing and administration).

Table 3.1 Clinical information derived from time and time management.

Time-related behaviour	Possible interpretation	Strategy
Patient is consistently late for session.	A therapy-interfering behaviour.	Discuss this in a direct and clear manner with the patient. Identify this as a pattern and be curious about the patient's conscious or unconscious reasons for this therapy-interfering behaviour.
Patient perseverates or is repetitive. Patient has difficulty following social cues, or seems to ignore clear statements around length of session time or cues that indicate the conclusion of a session.	May indicate cognitive or memory difficulties, or may be a symptom of a psychiatric disorder such as mania or hypomania. May also be indicative of problems with physical health, such as hearing.	Investigate further for relevant symptoms, through observation, and/or structured clinical interview.
Patient is tangential in content or pressured in speech.	May indicate a psychiatric disorder such as mania or hypomania, or may be symptomatic of a prodromal stage of psychosis.	Investigate further for relevant symptoms, through observation, and/or structured clinical interview.
Patient raises important points or concerns during the final few minutes of a session.	Avoidance of speaking about topic in session, which may be indicative of anxiety, worry, or shame.	Commence the next session by noting the topic. Invite the patient to note it first, then invite the patient to speak further about it.
Patient expresses risk of harm to self or others in the final minutes of the session.	Any expression of risk of harm to self of others must be sufficiently attended to.	Conduct a thorough risk assessment. This may require extending the session time and/ or contacting relevant crisis services, if necessary.

Therapists who have a natural disposition towards managing time well are still likely to need to make purposeful efforts around time with some patients or presentation, as issues arising from countertransference or other process issues may arise.

Agenda setting

An agenda is a plan of items to discuss in the therapy session. The agenda is set at the start of each session. This is an important element of many therapeutic modalities, but is more clearly explicated and communicated in some modalities, such as CBT.

The therapist models agenda setting in initial sessions. This is achieved by sign-posting content of the session. For example, in the initial session, the therapist may say:

> Today, our first session together, is an opportunity to hear from you about what's been happening in your life, and your current concerns. Later, we will have time to think about the goals of our work together. We will also look towards scheduling further sessions.

In all but the initial session, agenda setting can be a collaborative process. Allowing patients time and space to contribute to the agenda can be challenging for novice therapists, who may adhere strongly to a heavily scripted or overly detailed session plan. A balance must be maintained between the agendas of the patient and therapist; over time, therapists learn the clinical skills required to integrate both (Cozolino, 2004).

Agenda setting is succinct and direct. It can be completed in around one minute. This brevity ensures the session is focused on discussion of agenda items, rather than the agenda itself. A time allocation can also be given to each agenda item, in terms of minutes or proportion of the session. This can be based on a collaborative understanding of the importance of the agenda items and the therapist's informed judgement about the anticipated time to adequately discuss each item.

Some phrases may be useful in setting an agenda, such as:

> "How can we best use our time today?"
> "What's on your mind to chat about today?"
> "That sounds like an important thing to discuss; shall we put it on our agenda?"
> "Let's put that on our agenda to discuss."

"It seems we have a lot to discuss today. Can we prioritise these items to ensure we have a chance to cover the most pressing matters?"

Resist the temptation to enter into detailed discussion of items while setting the agenda; patients who tend towards giving overly verbose explanations of agenda items can be gently guided back to agenda setting by a brief statement, such as "Let's finalise our agenda first, then turn our full attention to talking about this."

Over time, the patient assumes responsibility for the agenda. This is an important process to ensure the patient is an active and engaged participant in sessions. Encouraging patients to contribute to the agenda also assists with the conceptualisation and understanding of their own presenting problem. For example, "I feel anxious" is a broad statement and a good starting point, but "I feel anxious about an upcoming exam" provides clearer direction and more targeted opportunity for an exploration and therapeutic intervention.

Most patients pick up the process of agenda setting efficiently and easily. Many will be familiar with the idea of agendas and the process of agenda setting through other contexts in the life, such as business meetings or lesson plans within educational settings, such as schools.

Some patients may not pick up the notion of agenda setting as easily as others. In these instances, the patient may find it difficult to contribute to agenda items, may ramble or become tangential while setting the agenda, or be overly ambitious in the amount or type of items to discuss in one session. In these instances, the therapist may need to be more directive in setting agenda items, providing feedback and guidance around the process. It may also be helpful to set agenda items as "homework", with patients asked to consider agenda items between sessions and present these at the start of the session (Beck & Beck, 1995).

Like any other therapy process, agenda setting is an important source of clinical information. Clunky agenda setting may indicate the need to revisit or revise treatment goals or treatment planning. It may also indicate the patient's tendency towards disorganised thinking. In this case, consider the notion of the therapy room as a microcosm of the patient's broader world and behaviour; that is, how this style of thinking may contribute to or perpetuate the presenting problem, and how others may experience the patient. For example, other people in the patient's life may share the therapist's annoyance or frustration at the patient's disorganised thinking or tendency towards being tangential; this is important clinical information that contributes to the formulation and adds to our understanding of the patient's life and experiences.

The "bell curve" rule

Many trainee and early-career therapists will recall the bell curve from behavioural science studies. A bell curve is a visual representation of data. The curve demonstrates a normal distribution, with most data falling within the mid-range. This is a representation of most human behaviour and traits, in which the majority of people and their behaviour falls within the "average" range.

The bell curve can also be applied to a therapy session. Most therapeutic content should occur in the middle of the therapy session. The build-up to the therapeutic content may contain a check-in regarding mood, update on homework, and agenda setting. Content is then discussed, with this taking up most of the session time.

A visual of this model can be kept in mind by the therapist during the session. Some therapists may find a more fixed visual representation helpful in order to apply it within the session; this may be a drawing on the therapist's notepad or note-taking device. The bell curve may also be used during session planning. Supervisees have reported benefit from plotting planned session content onto the bell curve, then referring to this during session in order to keep the session on track and to time. A representation of the bell curve model is presented in Figure 3.1.

Time management can be aided by ensuring new content is not raised towards the end of the session. This can help with finishing sessions on time, as new content or concerns will typically require discussion or exploration.

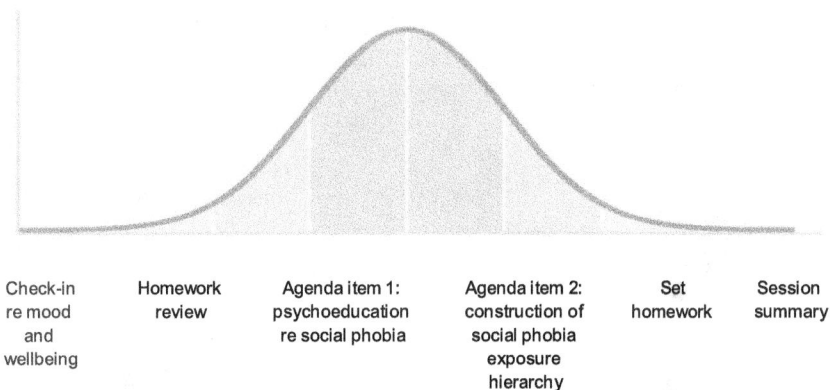

| Check-in re mood and wellbeing | Homework review | Agenda item 1: psychoeducation re social phobia | Agenda item 2: construction of social phobia exposure hierarchy | Set homework | Session summary |

Figure 3.1 Example of the bell curve rule applied to a therapy session.

Patients may also be distressed or unsettled by new content being explored, making it difficult for therapists to finish a session in a timely manner.

The bell curve model shows the intensity of the emotional content to be largely contained to the middle of the session. This way, the therapist has time to assist the patient in exploring and managing their emotional response that may arise from discussing the new content. This is in keeping with the notion that therapists should avoid finishing a session abruptly, as this increases the risk of the patient being in a state of emotional distress at the end of the session. A patient should never be left "high and dry"; containing therapeutic content to the middle of the session is one strategy to manage this.

Of course, not all human behaviour or traits fall within a normal distribution. There are always outliers. This also applies to therapy sessions. At times, sessions may skew in a positive or negative direction, either being top-heavy or bottom-heavy in terms of content and emotional intensity, respectively. Adopting a general template of the normal distribution can still be valuable in these instances and will help the therapist to be mindful of keeping to time and managing the content and emotional intensity of sessions. As in all aspects of therapy, flexibility is always preferable to rigidity.

Pie-chart strategy

Similar to the bell curve rule, session content can also be planned in accordance with a pie chart. In this model, session time is allocated to tasks or parts of the therapy session. Figure 3.2 shows how time may typically be allocated to each task, with a shorter opening section (mood check-in, homework review), leading to longer time for specific agenda items. The session is book-ended by a relatively shorter section of time at the conclusion of the session, allowing for session summary and/or homework setting.

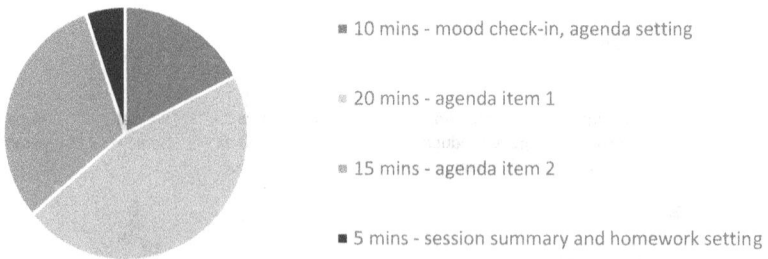

- 10 mins - mood check-in, agenda setting
- 20 mins - agenda item 1
- 15 mins - agenda item 2
- 5 mins - session summary and homework setting

Figure 3.2 Example of pie-chart strategy applied to a therapy session.

As per the bell curve model, the visual representation of a pie chart can be kept in mind during the session, drawn on the therapist's note-keeping device, or utilised during session planning.

Separating therapy and non-therapy tasks

Many therapists, especially those in private practice (see Chapter 11), are responsible for their own administration and other tasks related to patient care. This may include managing referral queries, correspondence with referrers and other third parties, report writing, billing or invoicing, and managing scheduling and appointments. This can be an effective and cost-efficient business approach for solo private practitioners. However, it is important to make efforts to separate therapy and non-therapy tasks, as blurring the two can impact time management.

In this context, therapy tasks refer to those that occur during time in the consulting room with patients. Non-therapy tasks occur outside of the consulting room, in the absence of patients. These may include administration, invoicing and billing, scoring psychometric tests, session planning, treatment planning, letter writing, report writing, correspondence with referrers and other health professionals, and appointment scheduling.

To this end, therapists should be careful to avoid "corridor conversations" before and after sessions. Corridor conversations refer to the discussion of clinical content outside of the therapy room. This may be in the corridor outside of the therapy room, in the waiting room, or in the reception area. Therapists should endeavour to keep therapy content inside the therapy room. Patients should be dissuaded from entering into conversation in the waiting room or other shared spaces. This is integral for patients' privacy and also demonstrates courtesy and consideration for others in the waiting room or shared space. Therapists can also model this by delaying questions such as "How are you today?" or engaging in other general conversation until the session commences. Remember, patients do not inherently know "how to do therapy"; some may benefit from a gentle reminder about keeping therapy content to the therapy room. This may be phrased as, "Let's chat about that when we start our session", or by providing nonverbal cues such as holding your own response to the patient's statement or query until in the therapy room.

Billing and invoicing can be managed by off-site reception or a virtual reception (VR). An alternative to outsourcing this task may be simply to create some virtual space between the therapist and administrative aspects of the therapy business, by having a separate "information" or "administration" email address operated by the therapist. Automatic payment systems common to many practice software management systems may also be used. While automatic billing can be effective and efficient, therapists should be aware of their ethical obligations regarding fair business dealings. This extends to pre-payment to sessions and automatic billing for sessions that are not attended or cancelled with insufficient notice.

Therapists should always make an effort to check the welfare of a patient who does not attend a session without prior notice (Barnett et al., 2014; Fairburn, 2008). This may include telephoning the patient or, in some instances, contacting the patient's next of kin. Ensure all efforts to contact the patient and all aspects of communication (including the patient's response) are clearly documented in the patient's file. Be wary of automatic credit card charges for non-attendance fees, or charging a card without the patient's explicit approval. An automatic charge to the credit card of a patient who is injured, incapacitated, or, in the worst-case scenario, deceased is likely to cause distress. This also reflects poorly on the therapist's professional and ethical conduct and could be reprimanded by a licensing board, professional body, or coroner.

★★

Sometimes, despite the best planning and efforts of the therapist, a session will run late or overtime. The therapist should make every effort to conclude the session as close as possible to time. Being overt about this with the patient ("I'm aware that we are running over time and need to finish up . . .") will help set a precedent around time-keeping.

The exception to this is in instances where there are concerns regarding risk of harm to the patient or to other people. A thorough risk assessment is always required when a patient expresses risk of harm to self or others. This may necessitate extending the session time, waiting with the patient until the arrival of a family member or caregiver arrives, or calling crisis or emergency services.

A short list of what *not* to do around time-keeping:

- Do not set an alarm to keep time in session.
  - An alarm is disruptive to dialogue.
  - The sound of an alarm, even those that emit a melody or tune, may be perceived as punitive, as alarms are typically associated with negative events.

- Do not extend session time for patients who arrive late.
  - Flag with the patient that the session will be shorter and that the session will conclude at the usual time.
  - Apply this rule consistently, even if your schedule might allow the session to be extended. Allowing extra time may set the expectation that this will occur in future sessions; concluding the session at the usual time encourages punctuality for later sessions.
- Do not attempt to squeeze more content into a shorter session.
  - Be realistic about the amount of type of content that can be discussed in a shorter session.

Concluding a session

Just as keeping time in session is the responsibility of the therapist, so is concluding a session in a timely manner. Many patients become accustomed to the flow of therapy and tend towards joining the therapist to keeping sessions to a duration of around 50 minutes. Some patients may not take to the structure as easily. Others will present new or important information at the tail end of a session. Colloquially called "49ers" (referring to the penultimate minute of a 50-minute session) or "door handle confessions", this may be considered an avoidant or therapy-interfering behaviour. That is, the topic or issue has been raised without ample time to consider it. The therapist should consider whether this may reflect anxiety about the topic, avoidance of discussing it, or genuine disorganisation on behalf of the patient.

> *"My supervisor modelled this for me. She would just end our supervision on time even if we weren't done. And I was okay with that."*

A patient should never feel rushed to finish a session. To this end, and in accordance with the bell curve and pie-chart strategies explored earlier, deceleration of the session should start well before the final minutes. This is especially true for patients who may tend towards being tangential or elaborative in their recall of information. Practical statements to assist with winding up a session when a patient has raised a new issue or continues to elaborate on an existing issue may include:

"This sounds like an important issue. We should devote appropriate time to it. Is it OK if we start our next session with this topic?"

"As we begin to talk about this, I'm just aware of the time . . ."

Nonverbal cues can be used to indicate the session is coming to a close. These may include glancing at the clock, picking up a diary (to indicate scheduling the next appointment), or, in some cases, standing up or motioning towards the door.

Some patients may not respond to verbal or nonverbal cues regarding finishing the session. In these instances, finishing a session will require more assertive statements or direct actions from the therapist. These may include:

"In the last few minutes of today's session . . ."
"We do need to finish up now . . ."
"We have come to the end of our time together . . ."
"We can pick up on that point first thing next session, but for now we need to wrap up . . ."

Core therapy skills

Core therapy skills include listening, verbal and nonverbal communication, the effective use of silence, building and maintaining rapport, and working with patients who may be difficult to engage. The best way to establish and maintain any of these core therapy skills is through practice. This can be achieved through a combination of activities:

- Reviewing video and audio recordings of sessions.
- Observing other therapists, either in person or via recordings. Sessions from many well-known therapists are available online or via the resource libraries of training institutes or universities.
- Feedback from patients. This may be verbal feedback, or ascertained via structured measures or questionnaires.
- Engaging in supervision. Both individual and group supervision will provide opportunities for activities, such as role plays, that will enhance core therapy skills.
- Engaging in therapy. Being the patient in a therapeutic setting allows exposure to new skills and facilitates vicarious learning.

Listening

Therapists have many tools at their disposal – psychometric measurement, assessment, diagnosis, and a plethora of treatment and intervention options – but the skill of listening should never be minimised or overlooked. Essentially, therapy is two people in a room having a conversation. It is one person listening to another.

Sometimes, patients and their stories will leave the therapist feeling overwhelmed and, in some instances, quite literally speechless. Some patients' lives and their stories can be difficult to comprehend. Their presentations can seem confounding or confusing. Many of their stories may seem stranger than fiction. Patients may have experienced or continue to experience unfathomable trauma. They may have engaged with a slew of mental health professionals over their lifetime and perhaps received inpatient treatment. They may be experiencing treatment-resistant depression, which has thus far not benefited from talk therapy, psychotropic medication, or other treatments such as electroconvulsive therapy (ECT). A patient may have a terminal health diagnosis, or may be grieving the loss of a loved one. There are some situations that therapists, even with comprehensive training and years of working with people, will find themselves throwing up their hands, feeling helpless and hopeless. Sometimes even therapists find it difficult to find the right words to say in response to another person's anguish. At these times, there may be only thing that can be done – listen.

Listening is arguably the most important skill a therapist can possess. Being heard is a primary need for patients. While therapists often think of therapy in terms of higher-order tasks of diagnosis and intervention, the primary reason for many patients presenting to treatment is, in fact, deceptively simple – for someone to listen, to get something off their chest, to debrief about life's stressors or an acute event. Essentially, most patients attending therapy want to be heard. No matter how skilled a therapist or how much training they achieve in advanced therapeutic modalities, this should always be kept in mind – the primary remit of patients presenting to therapy is to be listened to and heard.

> "And when you sit down in a room with another person who has come to you for help, park the theory in the back of your mind, and be present. First and foremost, be present."

A therapy session is a dialogue between two people. The therapist and patient engage in a conversation. But unlike a typical dialogue between two friends or acquaintances, which is reciprocal in that it (hopefully) has a somewhat equal focus on the needs and concerns of both parties, the dialogue of a therapy session is primarily focused on the patient.

The therapist's subjective thoughts and experiences are put aside for the duration of the session. This opens space for the patient to fully express themselves and their thoughts.

"Remember that you are a human being
interacting with another human being."

During informal dialogue, say a chat between friends, the reciprocity of conversation means that the split of "talking time" is typically 50/50. A therapy session entails a different type of conversation. The dialogue between a patient and therapist is typically weighed more heavily in the favour of the patient. In a therapy session, the majority of words should be spoken by the patient.

It is the patient's time to speak, and the therapist's time to listen. While every session differs, a general guide is that therapists should speak no more than 30–35% of the session time. The therapist will be speaking for a total of 15 to 20 minutes during a typical 50-minute session.

Attentive listening is often encouraged by telling people to "listen up" or "listen hard". Instead, therapists should embrace the notion of listening *softly*. That is, therapists need to soften to fully engage in listening. The esteemed Australian author Martin Flanagan (2016), renowned for his gentle writing about sports and sportsmanship, offers prescient advice and encouragement on listening:

> If you're quiet enough, quiet as a tree, people will camp beneath your branches and tell you stories you would never otherwise hear.

Therapists can adapt this information to the consulting room and therapy sessions. Be a sponge for the information that the patient is presenting. Take it all in and allow full absorption of the patient's words. For the duration of the therapy session, there is nowhere else to be, nothing else to do, no one else to listen to. Soften yourself; be open and receptive to whatever the patient may bring to the session.

Prior to the session, therapists can engage in strategies to best prepare themselves for listening:

- In the few minutes preceding a therapy session, do your best to bring your focus to the patient. Try to also keep in mind their presenting problem or what is likely to be discussed in session, if known.

- Ensure distractions during the therapy session are minimised. This may include turning off audible or visual notifications on computers or other devices, tidying your desk or workspace, or placing a "do not disturb" or "occupied" sign on the door.
- Prepare all necessary items and session materials prior to the start of the session. This may include water and glassware, printed information for psychoeducation, arts-and-crafts materials, equipment for specific modalities or interventions (such as EMDR equipment), copies of psychometric measures to be administered, and paper or other note-taking devices.
- Tasks that are cognitively taxing or distracting are best avoided in the few minutes preceding a session. These may include checking phone messages, responding to emails, or browsing social media.
- Introduce a ritual or practice to help calm your mind before a session. Strategies such as breathing techniques, a brief meditation, having a hot or cold beverage, or (my personal favourite) taking a few moments to look out the window.

Further strategies can be useful during the session:

- As best as you can, park anything unrelated until after the session. These can be attended to at the conclusion of the time with your patient.
- Be mindful of the general speed of your speech during sessions. Many people tend to speak quite quickly in conversation, which can leave the listener (the patient) feeling overwhelmed and rushed to respond.
- Therapists rapidly become accustomed to 50-minute conversations, but patients may find such long conversations fatiguing and overstimulating. Pacing speech and content is important to ensure all parties can engage in the session in a productive and useful manner.
- Count to three in your head before speaking in a session. This brief pause helps the therapist consider their words. This also models to the patient that conversations and responses during therapy sessions need not be rushed.
- Employ mindfulness in relation to your own listening. All therapists will sometimes experience concentration difficulties during a session. We may be fatigued after a poor night of sleep, or distracted by events in our own lives. Sometimes our minds wander to other tasks, our own to-do-lists, or our own concerns. This brief lapse of attention does not mean we are disinterested or dismissive of patients' experiences or what they are saying, but it may be a sign that we are trouble fully engrossing ourselves with listening. A mindful approach to this would include noticing the thought ("I'm noticing that my mind is wandering

or I'm having thoughts unrelated to the session") and providing a gentle reminder to bring your attention back to the room ("I will let those thoughts go", "those thoughts can be returned to later, after this session"). Instead, listen fully. It is perfectly acceptable to take a pause to consider your response and find the right words.

Practising listening skills in contexts other than work will also help generalise skills to the therapy room. Just as we ask patients to practise skills outside of sessions, therapists' practice of listening in their everyday lives can improve their in-session listening skills.

"Hone your mindfulness skills so you can stay present with your client even when your brain is going a million miles an hour."

Broader strategies are also useful to hone listening skills. These may include:

- Review video or audiotape of a session. Note down the cumulative minutes spoken by both the therapist and patient, respectively. Identify moments that were opportunities for you, as the therapist, to practise silence or allow the patient to speak further.
- Practise listening outside of the therapy room. Take a walk, sit on a train, visit an art gallery, sit under a tree, have a meal in a café or restaurant alone. And just listen. Note what you hear, what is said between people, and what seems to be left unsaid.
- Recall a time when you felt truly heard. What was special about that time? What did the listener do to facilitate your experience? Perhaps it was eye contact, their facial expression, body posture, verbal responses, or other factors.
- Listen to an audiobook, music album, or podcast – without multitasking. Concentrate only on the auditory stimuli.

Listening to and listening for

Therapists have a dual role of *listening to* while also *listening for*. Just as in any conversation, the therapist needs to *listen to*, in order to hear and make sense of the collection of words being spoken by the person with whom they are in dialogue. Therapists need to pay careful attention in order for the aural stimuli to be received, encoded, and stored; this is the memory process with which all behavioural science students will be familiar. Stimuli to which we are attuned has a higher chance of being encoded and stored correctly, thus increasing the likelihood it will be retrieved (remembered or recalled) when required. Therapists can usually follow with relative ease the *what* of a patient's story. That is, the patient's narrative, the main event of their story, their role in the story (protagonist, victim, bystander), the names and details of other people involved, and the chronology of events. Most therapists can also accurately detect the patient's emotional response that is associated with or seen as consequential to the story (for instance, happiness, sadness, shock, dismay, disappointment).

But therapists must also *listen for*. It is necessary but not sufficient for therapists to simply understand the facts of the patient's experience. The therapist needs to concurrently make sense of the information, while placing it within the formulation that is being developed and adapted with each new piece of information presented by the patient. Listen for the patient's tone of voice or inflection on certain words. Listen for missing information. Listen for repeated sentences, or for information that is reiterated or emphasised, perhaps by using the same words or synonyms. Listen for what is *not* said, for the space between words, for the gaps between phrases. Also pay close attention to the patient's nonverbal language, including posture (tense, relaxed), affect, facial expression (congruent or incongruent with affect), eye contact (avoidant, fixed), gestures of the hands and other body parts (fidgeting, still, catatonic).

"You must learn to listen, and listen closely."

The clinical skill of listening for while listening to develops over time. At first, the skill is a conscious one that requires intention, attention, and overt effort. Over time, however, established therapists find themselves integrating the skills, finding their capacity to hold and attend to different streams of information. Inherent to this is attending to important information while being able to identify and let go of superfluous information or details that do not contribute to the clinical picture or formulation of the patient.

Verbal communication

Decades of research findings support the notion of verbal communication being key to successful therapeutic outcomes. Appropriate verbal communication and well-phrased questions or queries can impact the direction of a therapy session, for better or worse. As a general rule, open-ended questions are preferable to closed questions; broad questions encourage the patient to give information they feel pertinent to the topic, rather than being directed by the therapist's notion of what may be a desirable or correct response. Verbal expression provides an opportunity for the therapist to convey their interest and attention to the patient, to demonstrate their understanding of the patient and their concerns, and guide the dialogue in a meaningful and therapeutic manner.

"Communication is the essence of our work. And connection. The central tools, they help you know you're on track."

Key aspects of verbal communication are summarised in Table 3.2.

Table 3.2 Key aspects of verbal communication.

Verbal communication	Example	Purpose or message conveyed
Minimal responses	"Hmmm", "OK", "I see"	Acknowledgement of patient's concerns. Encouragement for the patient to continue speaking.
Reflection	"You feel angry at Tom."	Emphasises a thought.
Paraphrasing	"Tomorrow is going to be a difficult day, with a full day of high-stake meetings and an after-work function."	Useful for summarising and rephrasing the patient's information. Can demonstrate the therapist's understanding of the patient's concerns.
Summary statement of content	"You attended the concert with Sarah and expected to travel home together, but she disappeared at the end of the evening."	Demonstrates understanding of the factual component of the patient's concern, without parroting or repeating their whole statement.
Summary statement of feelings	"You were really upset with Sarah for not waiting for you after the concert."	Demonstrates understanding of the affect component of the patient's concern, without parroting or repeating their whole statement.
Clarification	"Am I correct in thinking that things were OK between you and John, until the argument at Christmas dinner?"	Seeking confirmation of information. Checking understanding.

Table 3.3 Advanced aspects of verbal communication.

Verbal communication	Example	Purpose or message conveyed
Encouraging response	"Given what we've discussed, it seems you could manage that extra day of work that is being offered."	Providing feedback about the patient's readiness or capacity.
Challenging response	"You said you felt lonely and bored on the weekend, but also that you ignored messages from friends wanting to catch up?"	Increasing the patient's awareness or insight. Providing an alternate perspective.
Directive response	"As homework, I'd like you to attempt to complete the thought record exercise."	Setting a task.
Interpretation	"I wonder if you find that response from Tim especially frustrating, given that it's similar to how you've said your dad spoke to you."	Assigns a meaning to the patient's experience.

More advanced verbal communication includes questions and statements designed to prompt introspection, challenge the patient, provide interpretation, or provide direction. These are summarised in Table 3.3.

Just like any skill, the key to proficiency around communication is practice. This includes practising in and out of session, reviewing audio and visual recordings of previous sessions, and engaging in supervision and role plays which focus on communication.

Nonverbal communication

Therapy is typically thought of as a talking profession. It is true that words are a large focus of therapy work, but nonverbal information is arguably as important as that which is spoken.

Just as therapists are observant of patients' body language and draw inferences from nonverbal behaviour that add to our understanding and formulation of the patient and their presenting problem, patients are also impacted by therapists' body language and nonverbal communication.

At a bare minimum, therapists need to appear interested and engaged. Hopefully, this is always genuine, but even therapists are impacted by life events and sleepless nights, which may influence their levels of energy and enthusiasm. Therapists should adopt a stance of quiet calm and alert attentiveness (Cozolino, 2004). To this end, therapists must be aware of and alert to the message being conveyed to patients through their body language and nonverbal communication. Patients will be sensitive to signs of boredom or fatigue. This may pre-empt the patient shutting down or becoming resistant to therapy (whether consciously or unconsciously).

Be aware of body posture, body positioning, and physical movements. Table 3.4 presents a summary of nonverbal communication (Hackney & Cormier, 2012). The use of each should be considered carefully; overuse can make an otherwise significant gesture seem practised and disingenuous. It can be useful to notice the patient's body language and mirror (but not mimic) it accordingly.

The physical room in which the therapy session occurs also has implications for the therapeutic relationship. Therapy spaces are typically arranged so that therapist and patient are sitting adjacent to one another, rather than directly opposite. Computers or desks should be placed out of view of patients. The easiest and most effective way for a therapist to get a sense of the patient's experience of the consulting room is to take a moment to sit in the seat allocated to patients.

Table 3.4 Key aspects of nonverbal communication.

Nonverbal communication	Purpose or message conveyed
Head nod	Agreement Encouragement to continue talking
Learning forward in chair	Implies intensity and increased listening
Sitting with arms or legs crossed	Implies guardedness or lack of openness
Leaning back in chair	Disinterest
Open, relaxed posture	Openness, invitation to share
Soft smiling	Empathy, warmth, acceptance
Pensive facial expression	Reverence Recognition of the gravity or seriousness of the situation being discussed

Trainee or early-career therapists generally do not have a great deal of control over the consulting room in which they hold sessions. Training clinics tend to adopt a very basic style in terms of layout and furnishings. In these situations, think of the factors that can be controlled or temporarily modified – perhaps chairs can be moved to create a better sense of space between therapist and patient, or excess furniture such as desks or extra chairs can be moved to one side to create a more personable therapeutic space.

Established therapists usually have more input into the space in which they see patients. It is their workplace, where they spend significant time, and hence it comes to reflect their professional and personal style. Aspects of a good therapeutic space include comfort, professionalism, and emotional warmth. The structure should promote confidentiality, with noise control integral to any consulting room. A good therapeutic space is familiar and comfortable to both therapist and patient. Photographer Mark Gerald presented a fascinating photography series on the offices of psychoanalysts, capturing the vast individual differences in consulting rooms and further demonstrating the way in which a therapist's personality and therapeutic style can be conveyed by their work environment (Gerald, 2020).

Note-taking also presents an opportunity to consider nonverbal communication. Trainee and early-career therapists typically take copious notes. While this tends to alleviate the therapist's anxiety about missing any pertinent information, it can have the unintended consequence of diminishing the opportunities for connection and rapport-building between therapist and patient. This may include noticing facial expressions, making eye contact, and other potential points of nonverbal connection between therapist and patient. A notepad and pen, or another note-taking device, can act as a barrier between the therapist and patient.

Copious note-taking creates very "noisy" nonverbal behaviour. The patient may become hypervigilant on the type and amount of information being transcribed by the therapist; this may be taken as an indication of the therapist's interest in their concern, or viewed upon as a barometer of the severity or seriousness of the problem being described. More experienced therapists tend to take minimal notes during a session, or hold over their note-taking until after the session. Note-taking is covered in greater detail in Chapter 7.

The use of silence

Meaningful silence is always preferable to meaningless words. This is true in all conversations, but even more prescient in the context of therapy.

Novice therapists often fret about silence in sessions. This can lead to a rush to fill space, resulting in ill-considered or unnecessary statements.

This seems to be based on the assumption that silence is something to be avoided, and that therapy should involve a continuous dialogue without any space. But silence is both necessary and useful in therapy, just as it is during general conversation. Silence – whether for a short period of a few seconds for a longer time of several minutes – allows time for both the therapist and patient to think about a concept, ponder a question, or consider an appropriate response.

For the therapist, silence can also provide rich nonverbal data about the patient. During periods of silence, therapists have an opportunity to observe the patient's behaviour, mood, and affect. Does the patient seem elevated in mood, agitated, frustrated, fidgety? Have they appeared to "tune out" of the session? Might they be dissociative? Is their affect congruent with the subject matter being discussed? (For example, are they laughing when talking about a serious topic?) Do they seem to be using the time to consider a response, or are they having difficulty articulating their thoughts? This is rich clinical information that may be missed if a silence is prematurely interrupted.

Keep in mind that silence often feels longer in the moment; upon review of video or audio recordings, therapists often comment that a section of silence that felt elongated actually lasted for only a few seconds. This speaks to the importance of reviewing sessions and obtaining an objective perspective on the content and process of therapy sessions.

Sitting with silence is an integral therapeutic skill (Grosz, 2013). However, silence seems increasingly uncommon in our everyday lives, with the proliferation of electronic devices, headphones, and ever-increasing means of instant interaction and communication. Therefore, learning (or re-learning) to sit with silence is likely to take effort and time. This can be practised outside of the therapy setting, and then generalised into that context. For example, taking a walk without listening to music or a podcast (or if walking with a friend, allocating a few minutes of silence and resisting the temptation to talk), practising silent meditation, or simply sitting in silence for a designated period of time.

Some practical strategies can help the therapist and patient to ensure silence is adaptive and purposeful. These may be useful in situations such as when a patient is prone to extended periods of silence without a clear indication of when a response may be provided, or when the therapist feels they may rush too quickly into breaking a silence.

These may include:

• The therapist can resist interjecting by silently counting to a set number (such as 10 or 20) before breaking the silence.

- Saying to the patient: "Let's think about this for one more minute, then I'll ask you to share your thoughts".
- Prompting the patient by asking a "here-and-now" question, such as "Tell me, what's going through your mind right now?"

Building and maintaining rapport

Rapport refers to the mutual trust held between a therapist and patient. In a therapeutic relationship, rapport is the basis of the interpersonal contract between therapist and patient. It encompasses respect, trust, psychological comfort, and shared purpose (Hackney & Cormier, 2012).

Rapport is a necessary and sufficient condition for the development of a therapeutic alliance or working relationship. These three similar terms – rapport, therapeutic alliance, and working relationship – are sometimes used interchangeably; however therapeutic alliance or working relationship typically occurs after the initial establishment of rapport. Psychotherapy in the absence of therapeutic alliance or a working relationship is fruitless; both therapist and patient must be present, be engaged, and know what is expected of themselves and the other party (McWilliams, 1999). Decades of research points to the importance of therapeutic alliance as a determinant of optimal outcomes of psychotherapy. This finding holds true when other factors are accounted for, including presenting problem, patient symptomatology, and therapeutic modality. Further, the nature of the therapeutic alliance in the opening phase or initial sessions of psychotherapy is the best predictor of the outcome of that therapy; it is therefore prudent that the therapist must attend to the therapeutic relationship early and frequently (Gabbard, 2005).

Many years ago, a colleague told me their strategy to remind themselves of the importance of rapport. Next to the clock in their consulting room, out of view of the patient, was a small black-and-white photograph of Carl Rogers. Rogers was a much-revered humanistic psychotherapist, known for advocating a person-focused, non-pathologising, and non-judgemental approach to psychotherapy. Recognising the importance of rapport and the therapeutic relationship to treatment outcomes, Rogers coined the term "unconditional positive regard". Sometimes abbreviated to UCPR, this refers to the therapeutic benefit that is derived from the therapist demonstrating warmth and care for the patient. The inherent worth and dignity of each patient is recognised, independent of the therapist's subjective thoughts of the patient's behaviour, demeanour, or appearance. Sometimes it is easy to feel UCPR towards a patient; their personality or attributes may be similar to the therapist, or their experiences or presenting the problem may naturally elicit sympathy or empathy (Rogers, 1961).

Establishing or maintaining UCPR may be more challenging with some patients. Having a photograph of Rogers or writing UCPR on one's hand is a superficial strategy but offers a good reminder to the therapist of the importance of a warm and engaging therapeutic style. Beyond these surface-level strategies, the therapist should adopt an introspective position when reflecting upon problems with rapport or therapeutic connection. Consideration of transference and countertransference (see Chapter 8) will likely be key here. These concerns are best discussed in supervision (see Chapter 10).

The following questions may be used to prompt reflection around rapport building and therapeutic relationship:

- Is there a particular patient population or group of patients that I typically find challenging to engage with? For example, patients of a certain age or demographic (children, adolescents, older adults), or patients with a particular presenting problem?
- What is the indicator of poor therapeutic rapport? In other words, how do I know that there is a disconnection between the patient and me? Am I clock-watching, relieved when a particular patient is late to a session, or when a particular patient does not attend a session?
- Do I find myself experiencing worry, anxiety, or a feeling of dread in anticipation of seeing a specific patient?

There is no one set formula to build rapport or establish a therapeutic relationship. Importantly, it is an ongoing process, with the dynamic nature of therapy meaning that the relationship between therapist and patient will inevitably change over time.

Building rapport in a therapeutic relationship shares similarities to establishing any interpersonal interaction, such as a friendship or working relationship with a colleague. To this end, some useful strategies may include:

- Introducing yourself and your role.
- Implementing social skills. Be interested and attentive to the person sitting opposite you.
- Set some parameters for the therapy context. This might include ensuring the patient knows what is expecting of them and the session, such as the duration of the session.
- Notice nonverbal behaviour, and respond accordingly.

- Provide congruence with the patient's behaviour and interpersonal style. This might include an element of mirroring (as distinct from copying or aping) the patient's tone of voice, body language, or seating position. These small actions can demonstrate the therapist's awareness of the patient's affect, conveying empathy and understanding.
- Be authentic and genuine, while maintaining a professional stance.
- Be mindful of cultural factors that may impact rapport building. Be curious with the patient about how these may impact rapport and the working relationship. It is better to ask for clarity than to make assumptions about a patient's cultural background or experiences.

"Be more concerned with how you connect with patients."

The most reliable and straightforward strategy to build rapport is to be yourself. Aspects of a therapist's personality will shine through in their work. It is useful to integrate this into one's "professional self". Further, it is essential to demonstrate genuine regard for patients and attention and curiosity towards their interests. This does not mean feigning interest in activities or hobbies, but it might mean acquiring some general knowledge about activities or hobbies outside your area of interest. If you don't know something specific about a patient's hobby or interest – say, a sport or computer game – ask them. Patients are usually all too happy to explain their passion to an interested listener.

"Therapeutic rapport is important and can take time to grow.
Part of the process is building and nurturing this. Consequently,
some clients are going to take longer (and go backwards at times)
than other people (therapist, insurer, family members) would like
surrounding improvement."

Engaging and working with difficult patients

Some patients will be difficult to engage and challenging to work with. Analogous to Anton Chekhov's thinking about unhappy families, most patients who are easy to engage are easy in the same way, but difficult patients are all difficult in their own way.

A patient being difficult to work with is not necessarily a reflection of the therapist's skill or an indictment on their capacity to build rapport or establish a working relationship. Lack of rapport may be an indication of resistance on behalf of the patient. Resistance, in a therapeutic context, refers to conscious or unconscious strategies or behaviours the patient may use to block therapeutic progress (Gabbard, 2005; McWilliams, 2011). This may be in order to avoid change; thus, patients seek to preserve the status quo by avoiding engaging properly in treatment. Patient resistance to building rapport and establishing a therapeutic relationship may also arise from shame or difficulties with self-esteem or self-concept; this may inform the patient's belief about being undeserving or unworthy of receiving help, therefore precipitating lack of engagement or resistance towards attempts to build rapport and establish a therapeutic alliance.

Jeff Young (2023), an Australian family therapist, developed a novel and useful approach in working with reluctant patients. In his "No Bullshit Therapy" model, patients who are resistant to therapy are known as "therapy haters". Their counterparts, who seem to enjoy therapy and engage easily in the process, are termed "therapy lovers". These broad categorisations provide a helpful frame by which to consider the patient's aptitude for therapy and, importantly, provide a way forward to work with challenging patients.

"Therapy lovers" are often enjoyable for the therapist to work with. These patients are conscientious and punctual. They usually complete homework and other tasks. Rapport is easily established, and conversation flows freely. These "therapy lovers" are agreeable to suggestions and strategies and often demonstrate good motivation to change. But their agreeableness can also give way to a superficiality within sessions; both the therapist and patient may feel positive about the therapeutic interactions; however, one danger of this "warm and fuzzy" feeling coming from therapy is that sessions can become a conversation or catch-up without any actual therapeutic change being impacted.

Working with "therapy haters" brings more overt challenges. Arguably the biggest challenge here is the therapist's sense of self and professional identity. Even the most competent or experienced therapist is likely to feel demoralised and discouraged when working with reluctant patients.

Recognise that the source of a patient's resistance is unlikely to be a straightforward or direct reaction to any individual therapist. Therapists should not necessarily be personally or professionally insulted by a patient's lack of engagement; it is important to not mistake a patient's trepidation or anxiety for dislike of the therapist (McWilliams, 2011). Although some patients and therapists are a better therapeutic fit and an alliance is therefore more easily established, a patient's resistance is very rarely in response to anything about an individual therapist. Instead, therapists should be mindful of the dynamic at play (such as the therapist being viewed as a person who is powerful and imposing) and be wary of enacting patients' usual maladaptive coping strategies, such as stonewalling or leaving the relationship.

---

*"Be open, sensitive and curious about the
person who sits opposite you."*

Typically, patients mandated to attend therapy may demonstrate greater resistance to engaging in treatment. These patients may be attending therapy in order to fulfil a court order or directive from another authority. Other patients may not be mandated to attend therapy but are somehow otherwise obliged, such as at the behest of a parent, spouse, or other family member.

Young (2023) suggests the following strategies when working with "therapy haters":

- Acknowledge the patient's resistance to therapy.
- Identify the reason for the patient's resistance to therapy.
- Share with the patient your curiosity or working explanation about their resistance to therapy.
- Ask the patient how you might be able to work together to overcome the difficulties in the therapeutic relationship.
- Avoid jargon. Instead, use non-blaming, neutral language.
- Establish a clear mandate for the therapy work. That is, identify what work is to be done, and how it is to be achieved.
- Be direct, honest, and upfront about the constraints of therapy, such as what can or cannot be achieved.

Treatment plans and session plans

Treatment plans and session plans are essential, especially for trainee and early-career therapists. Without proper planning, treatment and sessions lack direction and may revert to a "chat" rather than a therapy session. Lack of planning is associated with suboptimal treatment outcomes and higher rates of patient drop-out. A lack of clear treatment planning is also cited as a deficiency common to therapists reported to licensing bodies or regulatory bodies for concerns regarding misconduct.

Treatment planning refers to preparation for the course of treatment. The time-limited and relatively brief therapeutic modalities utilised by most trainee and early-career therapists, such as CBT, lend themselves well to a treatment plan that is clear and structured.

Treatment planning should be informed by considerations about:

- The patient's presenting problem.
- Formulation.
- Appropriate therapeutic modality, with consideration of the therapist's training and competence.
- Psychometric measures that may be used to assess, evaluate, and enumerate the presenting problem.
- Appropriate goals of treatment.
- Anticipated length of treatment and/or number of sessions. This may be informed by therapeutic modality, preference of both therapist and patient, funding considerations, and organisational policy.

Session planning refers to the content and activities specific to each session. For some patients and for some presenting problems, session planning can be completed several sessions in advance. However, there is always a need for flexibility with session planning, to make room for variations within and across sessions.

Session planning may include:

- Focus/topic of each session
- Psychoeducation
- Formulation
- Administration of psychometric measure
- Specific activities for each session
- Homework tasks.

For example, Beck's (1995) seminal text *Basics and Beyond* provides a comprehensive model of the first and subsequent sessions for cognitive behaviour therapy. Barlow's (2021) excellent text provides a detailed breakdown of treatment planning and session planning for a number of clinical disorders, including post-traumatic stress disorder (PTSD), social anxiety, borderline personality disorder (BPD), mood disorders (including bipolar disorder), alcohol and substance use, and schizophrenia and other psychotic disorders. This comprehensive resource is useful for trainee and early-career therapists, together with experienced therapists seeking to learn more about treatment of specific presenting problems or disorders.

Many high-quality resources exist for both treatment planning and session planning. A few notable titles are summarised in Table 3.5, with a

Table 3.5 Useful resources for treatment planning and session planning.

Focus		Author
Therapeutic modality	Acceptance and commitment therapy (ACT)	Harris, 2019
	Cognitive behaviour therapy (CBT)	Beck & Beck, 1995
	Dialectic behaviour therapy	Linehan, 2015
	Psychodynamic psychotherapy	Gabbard, 2005
	Schema therapy	Young et al., 2007
Treatment of specific clinical disorders and presenting problems	Anxiety and mood disorders	Wells, 2011
	Anxiety and phobias	Beck et al., 2005
	Chronic health and medical problems	White, 2001
	Common clinical disorders	Barlow, 2021
	Eating disorders	Fairburn, 2008
	Family and relationship therapy	Minuchin, 2003
	Personality disorders	Sperry, 2016
	Post-traumatic stress disorder (PTSD)	Taylor, 2017

focus on presenting problems common to the work of trainee and early-career therapists.

Formulation

A formulation is a working hypothesis of the factors associated with the patient's presenting problem. This informs all therapy and clinical intervention. It is a personal representation of the patient and is unique to the patient and their circumstances. A formulation is a theory, informed by data from the patient (and potentially from other sources, such as family members or other health professionals), clinical judgement, and clinical knowledge. Importantly, a formulation represents the integration of the presenting problem with psychological theory (White, 2001).

An individual and tailored formulation should be developed for each patient. This is an essential process in understanding patients and their presenting problems. It also ensures an evidence-based approach to therapy and intervention. Working without a formulation is akin to a sailboat without a sextant; insufficient progress will be made, and circling the same water is highly likely.

A formulation is essential to good therapy. It informs the structure of therapy, in terms of overall treatment as well as content of individual sessions. Further, it enables the therapist to explore and explain the patient's concerns, and it provides an evidence base for planning and delivering treatment.

While formulation is an essential process for all patients, it can be especially helpful for patients with complex presentations, such as personality disorders (Sperry, 2016). For these patients, a formulation helps to organise and categorise information, providing a rationale for treatment and allowing change to be measured or evaluated over time.

The document shows the therapist's thinking and explains clinical judgement; this becomes especially important in the instance of a complaint against a therapist, with the therapist often required to demonstrate their understanding of the patient's presenting problem and provide evidence of treatment planning (Frankcom et al., 2016).

The "four P's" model is a popular method to construct a formulation. It takes into account the patient's past, present, and future in the context of the presenting problem. There is often interaction and overlap between these factors.

- Predisposing: factors relevant to the patient's vulnerability to developing or experiencing the presenting problem. For example, genetic or family history, personality traits, emotional regulation, self-esteem.
- Precipitating: factors and processes that pre-empt the patient's experience of the presenting problem. For example, role transitions and life changes, psychosocial stress, relationship problems.
- Perpetuating: factors and processes that maintain the presenting problem. For example, personality features, avoidant behaviour, home environment, interpersonal relationships.
- Protective: factors relevant to overcoming or treating the problem, such as social supports, past attempts to change, intelligence, psychological mindedness, motivation to change, professional support.

It is essential for trainee and early-career therapists to explicate this model with clear examples relevant to each of the "four P's". Over time, therapists internalise the conceptual framework of a formulation; established therapists will likely think about patients' presenting problems in accordance with the "four P's" without the need for explicit consideration of each of the four concepts.

Figure 3.3 offers a useful template. It is populated with information about a hypothetical patient, Heidi, a 23-year-old receiving treatment for anorexia nervosa.

PREDISPOSING	PRECIPITATING
- Maternal cousin diagnosed with bulimia. - Combative and verbally aggressive home environment, lack of open emotional expression. - Discordant relationships within family. - Parents' emphasis on weight and shape during childhood - Parents' comments on dieting and others' eating habits, including negative language to describe overweight or obese people. - Family focus on exercise and competitive sport.	- Difficulties with concentration and motivation, resulting in taking leave from study. - Difficulty establishing and maintaining social connections with other students. - Breakdown of relationship with long-term boyfriend. - Financial strain, resulting in decision to spend less money on food. - Marked increase in exercise (i.e., three-hour bike ride each day).
PERPETUATING	PROTECTIVE
- Continued emphasis on importance of weight and shape - Rigid rules around food. - Low self-esteem. - Interpersonal difficulties and lack of social engagement. - Leisure activities heavily focused on physical exercise.	- Good engagement with treatment, including individual and group sessions. - Increased insight into relationship with food. - Motivation to change. - Plans to return to study. - Support from mother and siblings. - Difficulty establishing and maintaining social connections with other students.

Figure 3.3 Worked example of a patient formulation.

A clear and concise formulation demonstrates a good understanding of the patient and the context of the development and maintenance of the presenting problem. This skill is especially useful for therapists working in fast-paced mental health environments, such as hospitals and acute psychiatric wards. In these settings, time is limited, and clinicians are expected to communicate important information in a clear and concise manner, usually at case conferences or patient handover between shifts.

This can be achieved by lifting one to two key sentences from each of "the four P's". For example:

> Heidi is a 23-year-old woman receiving treatment for anorexia nervosa. Heidi's long-standing thoughts about the importance of weight and shape were informed by early childhood and family experiences. Diet and exercise were valued and encouraged by Heidi's family members, particularly her parents. Recently, Heidi experienced several psychosocial stressors that precipitated significant weight loss, including falling behind with University studies and the breakdown of a long-term relationship. Heidi's disordered eating is maintained by rigid rules around food, frequent engagement in exercise as a leisure activity, and strong beliefs about her self-esteem being linked to weight and size. Heidi's good prognosis for recovery is strengthened by active engagement in treatment, medication compliance, increased insight, and support from her mother and siblings.

A formulation is dynamic. It requires frequent review and revision. This "reformulation" is conducted as the therapist's understanding of the problem as it develops, as further information is elucidated, or with changes to the presenting problem (White, 2001). While formulation is an essential guide to treatment, therapists must maintain flexibility and objectivity in thinking about a patient's formulation; patients' frustration at a therapist not understanding them or their problem is usually an indication of the therapist being unwilling or unable to maintain an open mind regarding formulation. Therapists should be wary of holding onto their formulation so tightly that it excludes the patient (McWilliams, 1999).

Sharing a formulation

The formulation should always be shared with the patient. The way in which a formulation is shared should be tailored to the individual patient, in terms of language and detail. The therapist should consider the formulation as the patient's information, with the therapists' role one of assisting in making sense of and organising the information. Inherent to this is the understanding that the patient is the keeper of their own information, and they have propriety over the information and how it is used and understood. Adopting this view makes the sharing of information not only important but obligatory.

Sharing the formulation also includes gaining the patient's input and feedback about the formulation. This typically occurs early in the therapeutic relationship, within the first few sessions. While this varies according to therapeutic modality and other factors such as presenting problem and patient symptomatology, two factors remain consistent – a formulation is a collaborative and dynamic concept.

It is also important to remember that therapists do not need to know every detail of a patient's life to conceptualise a valid formulation. Often, this is proffered by therapists as a reason to delay or withhold sharing a formulation with a patient. Patients are complex and have many facets to their lives; not all will be relevant to the current formulation. The formulation is based on relevant information about the patient's current clinical and background information in the context of the presenting problem. This hypothesis (or educated guess) will change over time, as the patient experiences or presents new information.

Sharing the formulation benefits the patient by encouraging collaboration and trust. It can also create necessary distance between the patient and their presenting problem by encouraging the patient to adopt a modicum of objectivity. This can be quite revelatory for patients consumed by their own thoughts about their situation, as they often have trouble "seeing the forest for the trees". Here, the patient is encouraged to be interested in their own problem and its solution, rather than being focused solely on their internal experience of the problem (Fairburn, 2008).

The formulation can be introduced with a brief statement. Remember that formulation is a clinical term; patients are unlikely to be familiar with this term, nor should they be expected to understand it. Plain, jargon-free language should be adopted, with an emphasis on collaboration, flexibility, and the dynamic nature of our shared understanding of a patient's experience.

> This is our current understanding of how and why this concern developed, and what is keeping it going. We may need to review or change this, as we get to understand this problem better. Your experience of this may also change in the future, which may also mean a change to our understanding of it.

When discussing the formulation with patients, ensure:

- Plain language is used, rather than technical terms or jargon. Avoid using the term "four P's", or any of the words predisposing, precipitating, perpetuating, or protective. Use language that is in keeping with the patient's understanding and style.
- Information is matched with the patient's level of understanding. This includes pacing the presentation of information.
- Emphasis is on the collaborative and dynamic nature of formulation. It is a *shared* understanding of the patient's concerns, rather than a monologue from the therapist.
- Initial focus should be on the main mechanisms and factors relevant to the formulation. Further information and detail can be discussed as therapy continues.
- Ask for feedback ("Have I got that right?"; "Does that sounds correct?").
- Check understanding by asking the patient to explain the formulation in their own words.

Further, it may be useful to draw a diagram or flow-chart of the "four P's". This is especially helpful with adolescent patients, or other patients whose literacy or educational level may present challenges to understanding complex verbal information.

The following example carries on from the previous information regarding Heidi.

> Heidi, it seems your ideas about weight and shape and the importance of dieting were formed early in your life, during your time growing up in the family home.
>
> Now, your sense of self and your self-esteem is closely linked to your weight and physical appearance. It also seems that recent difficulties with study and the break-up with your boyfriend, Sam, was especially distressing. In an attempt to gain some control at a time when very little was within your control, you became very rigid around food and exercise.
>
> I'm hopeful that we can work together towards meaningful recovery; you show a determination to make changes in your life, and I can see that you are motivated to engage in our sessions and also group therapy.

Ending a therapeutic relationship

All things come to an end, including therapeutic relationships.

One key to a good end to a therapeutic relationship is regular check-ins during the course of therapy. Progress towards therapeutic goals and the status of the therapeutic relationship should be discussed with transparency and in a collaborative manner. Frequent check-ins and the opportunity to discuss any perceived concerns about therapy and its progress will reduce the likelihood of a patient disengaging from therapy in an abrupt way or without explanation.

In short, there are three ways for a therapeutic relationship to end:

- In collaboration between the therapist and patient
- At the behest of the therapist
- Initiated by the patient

The length of treatment and number of sessions in a course of psychotherapy will vary greatly. This will depend on factors including therapeutic modality and the patient's presenting problem, and expectations of the workplace or organisation in which the therapist is employed. Funding and finances may also be a factor (whether therapy is funded privately, through insurance, or through another third-party arrangement).

Ideally, the end of the therapeutic relationship will be collaborative. One or both parties may initiate a discussion about progress towards treatment goals, and an agreement can be reached about an end point for sessions. Regular check-ins regarding progress throughout sessions about therapeutic goals can be helpful in broaching the end of sessions. The therapist can "plant the seed" about termination of sessions by alluding to the generalisation of skills or strategies to the patient's life after therapy has concluded.

"Given that this is our fifth session, it seems a good time to check in with the goals we set during our first couple of sessions."
"Let's allocate time today for a check-in on our progress."
"I am wondering how you are finding the process of therapy?"
"How are we getting along?"
"What are your thoughts about our sessions so far?"
"What are you finding most helpful about these sessions?"
"Do you think there's anything we could differently in these sessions?"

Some patients may resist the end of the therapeutic relationship. This may be in an overt way, where the patient will openly protest finishing sessions. Others may be less overt, with resistance coming through "acting out" or regressing in terms of symptoms and previous therapeutic gains.

Understandably, many patients experience therapy termination and the end of a therapeutic relationship as difficult or distressing. For many patients, the therapist represents a secure attachment and a meaningful relationship in their lives. This can be a novel experience for many patients and understandably becomes cherished. Given this, some patients may demonstrate a regression in behaviour or re-emergence of symptoms towards the end of sessions. Responding to this depends on several factors, including characteristics of the individual patient, presenting problem, treatment goals, and therapeutic modality or orientation. One strategy is to adopt a "here and now" approach, by acknowledging and working with the patient's resistance to ending therapy. In this approach, the therapist identifies the resistance and encourages the patient to reflect on the experience and consider whether similar thoughts or feelings have occurred at other times of change or at the end of other professional or personal relationships. Termination should then proceed as planned (Yalom, 2009).

Patients may be reluctant to initiate discussions about ending therapy. Remember, just like keeping time in session, we cannot assume that patients know how to "do therapy"; it is the role of the therapist to lead and educate the patient in the processes and etiquette of therapy, including termination.

Avoidance of talking about or enacting the end of the therapeutic relationship may lead to the patient disengaging in an ad hoc rather than planned manner. That is, they may terminate the therapeutic relationship by not attending a scheduled session, or by cancelling an appointment and declining to reschedule. This presents a missed opportunity; bringing the therapeutic relationship to a mutual end is an important skill, and one that provides modelling about interpersonal skills that the patient can generalise to other relationships and interpersonal dealings. Therapists can normalise the ending of a relationship, demonstrating to the patient that the discontinuation of a relationship can be non-conflictual, constructive, and a manageable emotional experience.

The termination of a therapeutic relationship is experienced by not only the patient, but also the therapist. This can represent a challenging time for therapists, during which they may feel a sense of sadness. Negative feelings may be more likely to arise at the end of a therapeutic relationship which was long term, was complex in some way, or came to a sudden or unexpected end. An adaptive approach to this involves talking with colleagues or seeking supervision. This is especially useful for therapists who find themselves ruminating about the end of a particular therapeutic relationship or specific patient; exploring this experience in a supervisory space may be beneficial in identifying the underlying mechanisms informing the therapist's affective reaction or response to the end of the therapeutic relationship (Hackney & Cormier, 2012).

It is normal for therapists to wonder about patients and their lives following the end of a therapeutic relationship. However, therapists should never allow their curiosity about a patient's post-therapy life to prompt them to contact the patient to check in on their well-being (except, of course, in instances of risk or when otherwise mandated to do so). Patients who require further assistance or wish to reengage in therapy sessions can contact the therapist; however, unless otherwise agreed upon, the therapist should not contact the patient.

Summary

- The second and subsequent therapy sessions provide an opportunity for the therapist to extend and expand upon the foundations of the first session.
- Time management is an essential skill for all therapists. Strategies to manage a 50-minute therapy session include agenda setting, good session planning and treatment planning, managing type and amount of content, and being mindful of the emotional intensity of the session over time.
- Core therapy skills include listening, verbal and nonverbal communication skills, and using silence in session.
- Most core therapy skills have their origins in everyday interactions. These can therefore be practised and developed in everyday life, and then further honed during therapy work.
- Rapport is a key factor in successful therapeutic outcomes. Rapport is important with all patients, but especially so when working with difficult patients or those who are hard to engage.
- Formulation, session planning, and treatment planning are essential "behind the scenes" therapy skills. Quality and consistency around these will benefit therapeutic progress.
- Ending a therapeutic relationship is an important task but can present challenges for both therapists and patients. There is no one-size-fits-all way of terminating sessions; however, the transition can be aided by planning, collaboration, and clear communication between therapist and patient.
- Trainee and early-career therapists benefit from focusing on mastering common therapeutic modalities, such as cognitive behaviour therapy. These provide an excellent foundation for the therapist to explore other therapeutic modalities later in their career.

Reference list

Adams, M. (2024). *The myth of the untroubled therapist* (2nd ed.). Routledge.

Barlow, D. H. (Ed.). (2021). *Clinical handbook of psychological disorders: A step-by-step treatment manual* (6th ed.). Guilford Press.

Barnett, J. E., Zimmerman, J., & Walfish, S. (2014). *The ethics of private practice: A practical guide for mental health clinicians.* Oxford University Press.

Beck, A. T., Emery, G., & Greenberg, R. L. (2005). *Anxiety disorders and phobias: A cognitive perspective.* Basic Books.

Beck, J. S., & Beck, A. T. (1995). *Cognitive therapy: Basics and beyond.* Guilford Press.

Corey, G., Corey, M. S., & Corey, C. (2024). *Issues & ethics in the helping professions* (11th ed.). Cengage.

Cozolino, L. (2004). *The making of a therapist.* Norton.

Denny, B. (2024, September 8). It's a nice idea, but more therapy won't fix our growing mental health crisis. *The Age.*

Fairburn, C. G. (2008). *Cognitive behavior therapy and eating disorders.* Guilford Press.

Flanagan, M. (2016). *On listening.* Penguin Books.

Frankcom, K., Stevens, B., & Watts, P. (2016). *Fit to practice.* Australian Academic Press.

Gabbard, G. O. (2005). *Psychodynamic psychiatry in clinical practice* (4th ed.). American Psychiatric Publications.

Gerald, M. (2020). *In the shadow of Freud's couch: Portraits of psychoanalysts in their offices.* Routledge.

Grosz, S. (2013). *The examined life: How we lose and find ourselves.* Chatto & Windus.

Hackney, H. L., & Cormier, S. (2012). *The professional counselor: A process guide to helping* (7th ed.). Pearson.

Harris, R. (2019). *ACT made simple: An easy-to-read primer on acceptance and commitment therapy* (2nd ed.). New Harbinger Publications, Inc.

Hart, A. (1985, March). Becoming a psychotherapist: Issues of identity transformation. In *Issues in the training and development of psychotherapists.* Annual meeting of the Eastern Psychological Association.

Linehan, M. (2015). *DBT skills training manual* (2nd ed.). Guilford Press.

McWilliams, N. (1999). *Psychoanalytical case formulation.* Guilford Press.

McWilliams, N. (2011). *Psychoanalytic diagnosis.* Guilford Press.

Minuchin, S. (2003). *Families & family therapy* (29th ed.). Harvard University Press.

Rogers, C. R. (1961). *On becoming a person: A therapist's view of psychotherapy.* Constable.

Sperry, L. (2016). *Handbook of diagnosis and treatment of DSM-5 personality disorders: Assessment, case conceptualization, and treatment* (3rd ed.). Routledge.

Taylor, S. (2017). *Clinician's guide to PTSD: A cognitive-behavioral approach* (2nd ed.). Guilford Press.

Wells, A. (2011). *Metacognitive therapy for anxiety and depression*. Guilford Press.

White, C. A. (2001). *Cognitive behaviour therapy for chronic medical problems: A guide to assessment and treatment in practice*. John Wiley.

Yalom, I. D. (1989). *Love's executioner and other tales of psychotherapy*. Basic Books.

Yalom, I. D. (2009). *The gift of therapy: Reflections on being a therapist*. Harper Perennial.

Young, J. (2023). *No bullshit therapy: How to engage people who don't want to work with you*. Routledge.

Young, J. E., Klosko, J. S., & Weishaar, M. E. (2007). *Schema therapy: A practitioner's guide*. Guilford Press.

Confidentiality   4

Confidentiality is a central tenet of therapy. Patients have a reasonable expectation that the information shared in therapy sessions will remain private. Confidentiality is a cornerstone principle for therapists; its importance is emphasised throughout education and training and is integral to rapport and trust within the therapeutic relationship.

"You'll take a bunch of stuff to your grave, that's part of the special commitment we make as therapists."

Being a therapist requires good keeping of secrets. Beyond supervision and peer consultation, there are few instances in which a therapist can discuss particulars of patients or their presentations. Therapists necessarily live their life in the background. There is little room for external praise or public recognition. Therapists need to become accustomed to intrinsic satisfaction being sufficient motivation and reward for their work.

Confidentiality may seem a simple concept. However, it can be a complex obligation, and it is the source of many ethical dilemmas. Decisions around confidentiality can greatly impact therapy, as demonstrated by the following hypothetical scenarios:

> A deceased patient's next-of-kin requests a copy of the patient's file, including all therapy session notes. The therapist is unsure whether this constitutes a breach of confidentiality.

DOI: 10.4324/9781003533030-4

A therapist overhears a fellow train passenger gossiping with a group of friends. The therapist quickly realises they are talking about a patient.

A relationship therapist sees the profile of a man they recognise to be a patient's husband on an online dating app. The therapist has a reasonable belief that his wife is not aware that her husband is using online dating platforms.

A therapist is talking with a colleague over coffee. They mention their latest patient is a "real handful" and gives details of the referral. The therapist realises that this is the girlfriend of a current patient.

A therapist receives an email from the stepmother of a 14-year-old patient. The stepmother details aspects of the patient's life of which the therapist was not previously aware, stating her concerns that her stepchild has not been truthful in sessions. The stepmother asks the therapist to inform the patient of the correspondence.

A therapist receives a request from a lawyer for a patient's file. The therapist has not seen the patient for several years. The letter is accompanied by a "release of information" form signed by the patient.

Confidentiality and the therapeutic relationship

Therapy is a point of curiosity for many people. In social settings, therapists are often asked questions about their role. Some inquisitive strangers may seek mental health advice, either for themselves or a loved one. Others may push for details of the "craziest" patient or most bizarre presentation a therapist has encountered. Therapists should not entertain these questions; both present risks to confidentiality.

Humans are social creatures. It can feel natural to share the details of our lives, including details of our work, with others. Therapy work is genuinely interesting; and patients' stories are often stranger than fiction. But patients and their experiences are not fodder for gossip, nor content for dinner party conversations. Patients' information does not "belong" to therapists, and as such, therapists have no right to share patients' stories. Therapists must not exploit or capitalise patients' information for social gain or other reasons.

Even therapists cognisant of their responsibilities around confidentiality can find themselves being seduced by requests to share information. Therapists are human, and their egos are naturally flattered by others' being interested in their work (Cozolino, 2004). But therapists who find themselves talking about work within their social life – whether therapy anecdotes or details of specific patients or presentations – would likely benefit from exploring their experience of countertransference, either through supervision or personal therapy (see Chapter 10).

> *"It's essential that you feel you're a good-enough*
> *vault for your patients' information."*

The nature of a therapist's work differs from many other occupations, in that therapists cannot debrief about their professional dealings with a spouse, acquaintance, or friend. These restrictions can be difficult for non-therapists to understand, and as such, some people may try to push therapists to break confidentiality by asking details of patients or the content of a therapy session. It is imperative that the therapist respects the confidentiality of their patients. This includes social conversations with other therapists; peer consultation with other therapists is appropriate, however general gossip is not.

> *"You might have a good story about a patient for your friendship*
> *circle, and even if it is completely de-identified, what perception*
> *are you portraying? Are you giving the public the perception that*
> *psychologists dine out on their patients' interesting lives?"*

Limits of confidentiality

Patients have a reasonable expectation that the information shared with therapists will be held confidential. However, confidentiality in the therapeutic relationship is never absolute. Any material generated by therapists in the course of their work may eventually be accessed by a person other than the therapist, including the patient or a third party such as an insurer, or accessed in the context of legal proceedings. The process of informed consent (see Chapter 2) is essential to educate patients about confidentiality and its limits.

Generally, information shared in therapy is held confidential, except for the following conditions:

1. Consent is provided by the patient to share information.
2. Where required by law.
3. Where failure to disclose information may place the patient or another individual at serious and imminent risk.

Patient requests for information

Patients may request access to their own information. While rules around privacy and health records differs by jurisdiction, provisions for patients' access to their own information are made under privacy laws. As such, therapists should write notes and other documents in professional language and in a manner that is adequately comprehensive, but remains sufficiently accessible to others.

Therapists should not refuse reasonable requests from patients to access their information (Pelling & Burton, 2019). Privacy laws provide for patient access to information; however, there are several options for the dissemination of this material. "Raw information", such as session notes, may not be easily comprehendible by patients, despite therapists' best efforts to write these in plain language. An alternative to reading session notes is for the therapist to offer a report or written summary of the patient's engagement in therapy. The therapist may offer to sit with the patient during access to the file, in order to answer any queries or to provide further explanation or context to the written information.

Patients may also request others to have access to their information. This may include a third party, such as another health professional, lawyer, or family member. Privacy laws also apply to these requests, and as such, therapists should not refuse a reasonable request for access to information. However, the therapist must ensure that the patient has provided sufficient consent and is truly informed about the nature of the release of information. In some instances, patients sign broad "release of information" forms at the encouragement of legal representatives; some patients may not be fully cognisant of the information being requested on their behalf. Prior to releasing any information, therapists should contact the patient to clarify their understanding of the request.

> *"Be mindful of the scope of confidentiality breaches.*
> *A patient may give you permission to get their spouse's*
> *perspective on their current functioning; this doesn't necessarily*
> *give you permission to disclose facts about their early life that*
> *you may have learned in therapy."*

Children, families, and other vulnerable patients

Informed consent, including that for confidentiality, can be provided only by competent adults. Children and other vulnerable individuals (which may include people with cognitive impairment or an intellectual disability, or those whose competence may be impaired due to a psychiatric condition) still have a right to confidentiality. However, considerations around this can be more complex. Typically, informed consent is obtained from parents or caregivers of these individuals; however, assent from the individual can also be sought. An explanation around confidentiality must be appropriate to both age and context. Like informed consent, assent is an ongoing process, with concepts of privacy and confidentiality revisited as required throughout the therapeutic relationship.

The concept of a "mature minor" attracts some discussion in therapy circles. In truth, there is no arbitrary cut-off point or age where an individual transitions from a child to an adolescent, or to an adult. This is a point of interest for therapists working with adolescents, particularly when a question arises about whether a parent should be informed of a disclosure made during session. In such instances, therapists should be encouraged to adopt clinical rather than emotive thinking, putting aside their personal views which may be impacted by their own experiences as a parent or caregiver. Instead, clinical decision-making should be applied. Revisit informed consent and/or assent, and provide clear communication to all parties. If appropriate, discussing the decision-making around this with the patient can be useful from a therapeutic perspective, as it is likely to provide information about the patient's thoughts and feelings about family dynamics and communication (McCool, 2024).

Mandatory reporting (duty to warn)

In some jurisdictions, therapists are mandated reporters. This means it is compulsory for therapists to disclose information if they have a reasonable belief of a serious threat to life, health, or safety. The concern may be related to a specific individual or group, or more broadly to public health and safety.

Related to this is the concept known as "duty to warn". The Tarasoff case is often cited to illustrate the important role of therapists in protecting individuals and the public from potential harm. In 1969, University student Prosenjit Poddar informed his campus counsellor of his intention to kill Tatiana Tarasoff, a woman about whom he had developed an infatuation. The therapist disclosed the information to his colleagues and alerted campus police; however, the therapist's concerns were not adequately followed up by campus police and administrators, and Poddar killed Tarasoff.

Since the Tarasoff case, several other high-profile court cases have also focused on the role of therapists in disclosing information when necessary to protect individuals or the broader public from harm (Corey et al., 2024). Laws around mandatory reporting differ within and between jurisdictions. Distinct rules also apply according to profession; for example, in Australia, psychologists are deemed mandatory reporters, together with other professionals such as medical doctors and teachers (Australian Psychological Society, 2020). It is incumbent upon all therapists to know their responsibilities regarding mandated reporting. Being unaware or uninformed of one's responsibilities is not sufficient and not considered a valid explanation by registration boards or licensing boards in the case of inaction or negligence by a therapist.

Therapists are not expected to predict the behaviour of their patients, including violent behaviour. It is not the role of the therapist to make conclusive statements or judgements. Rather, it is the role of a therapist to report the facts of a situation as known to them, and for relevant authorities to then assume the role of presenting the facts of a situation as known to them.

Duty to warn and mandated reporting apply to the therapist's patients, in addition to other individuals and the general public. Reportable abuse may include physical, sexual, emotional, or financial abuse, or neglect/ abandonment. Therapists may also need to consider safety implications for patients who fall outside of their usual scope of practice or area of competence, such as families, children, or other vulnerable groups such as the elderly or people with disabilities. In this instance, appropriate supervision or guidance should always be sought.

"Regardless of whether I am talking with clinical or admin staff, how much information do I need to provide in order to achieve what I need to? Am I disclosing irrelevant details for the task at hand?'"

Legal requests and subpoenas

Therapists may receive requests for information about patients from lawyers and other professionals within the legal field. This can be an anxiety-provoking experience for therapists, but it is useful to remember that a request for information from a therapist – whether a legal request or a subpoena – is about the patient, not the therapist. The therapist and their work are not on trial. A request for information does not mean the therapist's work will be scrutinised.

Above all, therapists should keep their patient's well-being at the forefront of their mind with any legal request or subpoena process. It is usually in the patient's best interests for therapists to respond in a professional and efficient manner to all matters related to legal proceedings. Any individual who has experienced involvement in legal proceedings (whether of a professional or personal nature) will appreciate the benefit of all parties acting in a professional and efficient manner.

Much of the anxiety from novice therapists comes from lack of clarity around understanding the purpose of legal requests and subpoenas. It is important that therapists understand the distinction between legal requests and subpoenas. While there is overlap between the two, each carry distinct responsibilities for therapists.

A legal request usually comes directly from a legal representative, such as a lawyer or a legal firm. The legal representative making the request may be representing the therapist's patient or may be acting for another party. Rules and procedures regarding release of information to legal representatives vary between jurisdictions and may depend on the type of legal matter under consideration. As such, therapists should always consult relevant legislation to ensure compliance with their professional and legal obligations. Supervision and access to legal advice should also be sought. Professional bodies provide current information regarding this and typically provide advisory services to members around release of information (Australian Psychological Society, 2016).

A subpoena is a court-ordered request for information or documents. A representative of the court (typically a judge or judicial registrar) has approved a request made on behalf of a legal representative involved in a patient's legal case. A subpoena will include a clear statement of the actions required from the therapist. These usually include providing a copy of the patient file or being required to appear in court to provide information.

Therapists *must* comply with a subpoena. Not doing so may result in a breach of court; this is a serious offence, with possible consequences ranging from a fine to a custodial sentence. Never ignore a subpoena. Receiving a subpoena may be anxiety-inducing, particularly for novice therapists; however, avoiding or ignoring a subpoena reflects poorly on the therapist's professional standing and will almost certainly lead to greater difficulties than those that would arise from complying with a subpoena.

An overview of the process for complying with a subpoena is provided in Figure 4.1. The information provided is adapted from the Australian Psychological Society's guide on managing legal requests and subpoenas (Australian Psychological Society, 2016).

The patient record or specific documents that have been requested must be contemporaneous (Frankcom et al., 2016). The documents must be an

Check validity	A subpoena carries a court stamp, seal, or judicial signature.
	Legal requests can appear similar in presentation and formatting, but will not carry an official court stamp, seal, or judicial signature.
Check return date	Requests must be accommodated within set timeframe.
	Contact the court immediately if the timeframe is not able to be met.
Check requirements	A subpoena typically asks for production of information (such as patient records) and/or for the therapist to attend court to provide evidence.
Inform patient, where possible	Therapists should make every reasonable effort to inform patient of the subpoena.
	Note that inability to contact patient is not a valid reason for non-compliance with a subpoena.
Object to producing documents, if necessary	Therapists with a reasonable belief that some or all information should not be provided must follow the procedure deatiled in the subpoena.
Comply with requirements	This may include production of documents (typically sent via registered mail or secure online portal) and/or attendance at court.
Claim costs	Compensation may be payable for production or documents or attendance at court.
	Fee schedules for these activities are published by professional bodies.

Figure 4.1 Process for complying with a subpoena.

accurate and timely reflection of the therapist's interaction with the patient. Never amend a record that has been requested as part of a subpoena.

In some instances, a therapist may reasonably believe that certain information contained in the patient file should be withheld from legal proceedings. This may be because information is deemed irrelevant to the legal matter, or that disclosing information (such as names, events, or addresses) may lead to a person being at risk of harm. Other information, such as psychometric test materials that are covered by copyright law, should also be excluded. Prior explicit approval must be provided by a court to redact any information. Therapists should communicate their concerns promptly in writing to the relevant person listed on the subpoena. Redacting information without prior approval may represent a breach of court. The therapist should immediately notify the issue of the subpoena in the instance of any information not being able to be provided (perhaps due to a missing file, or difficulties or delays in accessing archived records).

Managing the therapeutic relationship during confidentiality breaches and information disclosures

Rules around confidentiality protect the trust an individual has about their personal information being kept private. Therapists sometimes report reluctance to disclose information due to concerns around potential impact on the therapeutic relationship. But the requirement of a therapist to breach confidentiality by disclosing information need not necessarily cause a rupture in the therapeutic relationship. Where possible, and when safe to do so, the therapist should endeavour to inform the patient of the need to breach confidentiality by disclosing information. In some instances, the patient may be relieved that their concerns are being taken seriously, and that action is being taken on their behalf.

The following scenario, as illustrated in Figure 4.2, demonstrates one way of protecting the therapeutic relationship within a therapeutic relationship.

> Hannah, 35 years old, has been attending therapy sessions for parenting support in the context of difficulties within her marriage. She reports her husband to be a heavy drinker and has expressed concerns about his alcohol use around their pre-school children. Hannah recently told her therapist of a specific incident in which the children were left unattended for several hours when in their father's care. The children were distressed when Hannah arrived home from work. Hannah reported that when she reached her husband via telephone, he sounded intoxicated and could not provide his location.

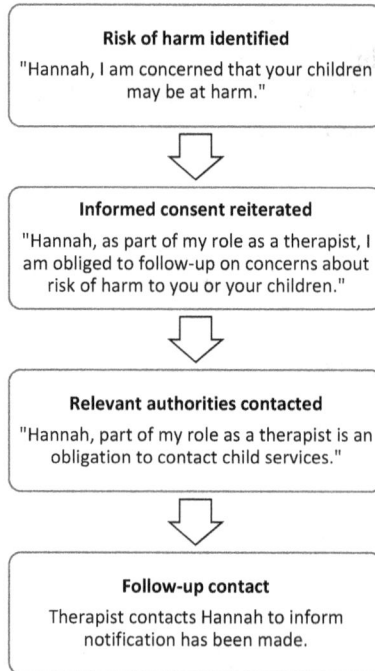

Risk of harm identified

"Hannah, I am concerned that your children may be at harm."

Informed consent reiterated

"Hannah, as part of my role as a therapist, I am obliged to follow-up on concerns about risk of harm to you or your children."

Relevant authorities contacted

"Hannah, part of my role as a therapist is an obligation to contact child services."

Follow-up contact

Therapist contacts Hannah to inform notification has been made.

Figure 4.2 Informing patients of need to breach confidentiality or disclose information.

Practical strategies to manage confidentiality

Prevention of a confidentiality breach is better than any attempt to cure it.

Practical strategies can be adopted to minimise the risk of confidentiality breaches. Consulting rooms should be adequately soundproofed. Patients whose volume of speech is particularly loud may need to be encouraged to be mindful of the capacity for others to hear their conversation, both in terms of their comfort and that of others who may overhear the therapy conversation. Avoid "corridor conversations" and minimise interactions in shared spaces such as waiting areas. It can be distressing for patients to recognise or be recognised by other patients. Incidental encounters may be minimised by staggering appointment wait times, or asking patients to arrive near to their appointment time.

"Confidentiality 'slips' are most likely to occur in subtle and casual ways. Am I debriefing, or am I gossiping? Does this need to be discussed now, or can it wait until my next supervision session?"

Online behaviour

The proliferation of the Internet and online communication has impacted many traditional concepts of therapy. No longer is therapy necessarily a face-to-face interaction, nor are files paper-based and stored in one location.

Most therapists now conduct at least part of their practice remotely, via telehealth or other video platforms. Notes and records are usually stored electronically. These advances in technology have made many aspects of therapy work convenient and accessible; however, with these benefits come new risks to confidentiality. Therapists must ensure all online communication is secure and encrypted, and that electronic records are adequately safeguarded (see Chapter 7 for further information).

An increasing number of therapists use social media and other online tools for professional purposes. The tenets of confidentiality apply to these contexts. It is never appropriate to disclose specific patient information online, even in private forums such as those designed for peer support.

Summary

- Confidentiality is a central tenet to therapy. It is the basis of the trust inherent to therapeutic relationships.
- Patients can reasonably expect their information to be safeguarded by therapists. However, confidentiality in therapy is not absolute. Patients are made aware of this through the process of informed consent.
- Therapists are required to disclose information under certain conditions, including when a patient has provided consent to share information, where required by law, in instances of serious or imminent risk.
- Where safe and feasible to do so, patients should always be informed of a therapist's need to break confidentiality or provide information to a third party. This can help maintain a good therapeutic relationship.
- Therapists are sometimes called upon to provide information for legal proceedings. This can be in the form of legal requests or subpoenas. Therapists must be cognisant of their rights and responsibilities related to both legal requests and subpoenas.
- In terms of confidentiality, prevention is always better than cure. Strategies may include ensuring noise control in consulting rooms, managing shared spaces such as waiting areas to avoid unnecessary patient interactions or social conversations, and being aware of privacy on online platforms and online tools such as social media.

Reference list

Australian Psychological Society. (2016). *Managing legal requests for client files, subpoenas, and third party requests for psychological reports*. Australian Psychological Society.

Australian Psychological Society. (2020). APS ethical guidelines for reporting abuse and neglect, and criminal activity. *InPsych, 42*(6).

Corey, G., Corey, M. S., & Corey, C. (2024). *Issues & ethics in the helping professions* (11th ed.). Cengage.

Cozolino, L. (2004). *The making of a therapist*. Norton.

Frankcom, K., Stevens, B., & Watts, P. (2016). *Fit to practice*. Australian Academic Press.

McCool, S. (2024). *Working with child and adolescent mental health: The central role of language and communication*. Routledge.

Pelling, N., & Burton, L. J. (Eds.). (2019). *Elements of ethical practice: Applied psychology ethics in Australia*. Routledge.

Professional boundaries in therapy   **5**

All people, including therapists, have a range of relationships. This may include social acquaintances, friendships, collegial relationships, and romantic or intimate partnerships. Some are transient, others long-term, with a few lifelong. These interpersonal relationships are typically reciprocal; information is shared within an open dialogue, and contributions are generally expected from each person. Focus may favour one person at times, such as when a friend is experiencing a difficult time or a significant life event, but generally there is ebb and flow in conversation.

Therapeutic relationships differ from these typical relationships in several important ways. A therapeutic relationship is a professional association between a therapist and patient. Most importantly, the reciprocity inherent to other interpersonal relationships is largely absent from therapeutic relationships. Reciprocity, defined as an exchange for mutual benefit, might be demonstrated by statements such as, "Oh, me too!", "I had that same experience, let me tell you about it . . .", or "Wait until you hear what I went through at that same place!" These statements are usually suitable for a conversation with a friend, but not during a therapy session. Therapists are not friends, and friends are not therapists.

The focus of the information in this chapter is understanding and managing boundaries and therapeutic relationships in a manner that is consistent with professional and ethical standards expected of therapists. Considering this information in conjunction with other therapeutic processes, such as transference and countertransference (see Chapter 8), will promote a more complete understanding of boundaries in relation to therapeutic relationships and therapeutic treatment.

DOI: 10.4324/9781003533030-5

Boundaries

Boundaries represent the parameters of a therapeutic relationship. Boundaries are integral to provide framework, structure, and expectations to the relationship between a therapist and patient. Rules for the process and content of therapy are informed by boundaries. These provide the therapist with a reference point and direction to manage interactions with patients.

Boundaries are necessary in any profession in which there is a power differential between provider and consumer, such as within a therapeutic relationship (Yalom, 2009). Clear boundaries provide safety and containment for patients (Gabbard, 2005).

Therapists must be cognisant of both *boundary crossings* and *boundary violations*. Boundary crossings (also known as *boundary transgressions*) are actions which are deemed appropriate in the clinical context and are therefore considered to be professionally and ethically acceptable. In contrast, boundary violations are actions that are inappropriate in a clinical context. These may be harmful or exploitative of the patient.

Sometimes, the grey area between boundary crossings and boundary violations can be challenging for therapists to interpret. This may be especially true for trainee and early-career therapists, who are learning the process and skills required to deliver therapy while also considering ethical and professional aspects of practice. Therapists must work proactively to strike a balance between conducting effective therapy while being mindful of both boundary crossings and boundary violations.

"Even as you need to develop a stance that some might call professional distance. I think of it more as a type of composure. A way of saying: Here I am. My door is open. You're welcome to step inside and tell me what ails you. Together we can think about how best to make things easier for you."

Outside of therapy, the term "boundaries" is frequently used in everyday language and conversation. This is a different context to the professional understanding and application of the term. In common parlance, "boundaries" typically refers to a person needing space or setting parameters around interactions with another person or group of people, primarily to protect one's own well-being. The key point of difference is that when used by lay people or non-therapists, the focus of the term is on protecting the self; for therapists, however, boundaries represent a professional responsibility and are put in place in order to protect another person (i.e., the patient).

It is incumbent upon the therapist – not the patient – to establish and maintain appropriate boundaries. The ease of this varies across patients and presentations. Patients with personality disorders, attachment-based disorders, or other complex presentations can present particular challenges in establishing and maintaining professional boundaries within a therapeutic relationship. The nature of these presentations typically involves inter-personal difficulties, or insecure or disorganised relationship patterns or attachment styles. "Testing the limits" (i.e., pushing boundaries) of personal relationships can be common to these presentations. This is likely to also play out in professional relationships, such as with a therapist; whether knowingly or unknowingly, the patient may breach professional boundaries and seek to disrupt the power differential inherent to a therapeutic relationship. This may include flirtatious or sexual behaviour, excessive gift-giving, bartering for services, or assuming privileges such as extra session time or access to last-minute appointments. Some patients may perceive their relationship with the therapist to be "special" and therefore somehow transcendent of professional boundaries that apply to patients (McWilliams, 1999; Sperry, 2016). Seminal research with therapists who have engaged in sexual relationships with patients demonstrated the importance of respecting and maintaining the power differential between therapist and patient; neutralising the power dif-ferential towards an equal relationship (i.e., not acknowledging the different status of therapist and patient) was identified as a key factor (McNulty et al., 2013). Other significant risk factors included therapists' minimising the mental health concerns of the patient and not engaging in sufficient supervision.

> *"Issues of boundaries and ethics often arise when people are not aware of their countertransference."*

Boundary crossings

Boundary crossings are actions that constitute a clinically appropriate course of action. These are consistent with the patient's clinical history and thera-peutic goals, and they are informed by the therapist's clinical judgement. Also referred to as boundary transgressions, boundary crossings are deemed appropriate by both therapist and patient (Barnett et al., 2014). Factors such as cultural considerations, patient presentation, and therapeutic modality also influence decisions around boundary crossings.

The actions comprising a boundary crossing may seem unprofessional or unethical when considered out of context or without appropriate detail. For example, self-disclosure – where a therapist shares personal information about themselves with a patient – may seem contrary to the teaching and application of therapy. However, in some circumstances, self-disclosure may have therapeutic value. A therapist may share a personal anecdote or preference (e.g., their preference for a food or appreciation of a style of music) with a patient, perhaps in the context of building rapport or normalising a behaviour. Sharing information regarding food or music is unlikely to be viewed as a boundary violation by the patient or therapist.

"Would I feel comfortable disclosing in supervision any action or comment made in the privacy of the therapy space? If the answer is no, you almost certainly have crossed a professional boundary, and for a reason that is difficult to justify."

Trainee and early-career therapists are typically mindful of boundaries. They are especially cognisant of actions and behaviour that clearly represent boundary violations, such as socialising or engaging in any sexual activity with patients. Less clear are boundaries around touch, receiving gifts, and self-disclosure.

Physical contact encompasses a broad range of actions, including touch. Generally, touch is considered to be inappropriate and unnecessary within talking therapies, and as such this is clearly stipulated in codes of conduct. However, some touch may be appropriate, such as a handshake during an initial greeting. When sparingly used, other touch may provide reassurance or comfort to patients, such as a further handshake or light hug. Therapists should avoid touch when in doubt or in situations in which touch may be misinterpreted, even in instances initiated by the patient. Any physical contact needs to be considered in the context of professional boundaries, cultural appropriateness, and therapeutic utility.

Some patients will seek to express their gratitude to therapists through the giving of gifts. This presents a common grey area in terms of boundaries. Typically, codes of conduct and ethical guidelines stipulate that receiving gifts is dependent upon the significance of the gift in terms of size and expense. In considering whether to accept a gift, the therapist must be cognisant of knowingly or unknowingly setting up expectations around giving and receiving gifts as part of the therapeutic relationship. Gifts should never be a proxy for some or all of the session fee. Small gifts such as a box of chocolates or a book at the conclusion of a therapeutic relationship or at the time of a culturally significant date, such as Christmas, is appropriate and typically presents no ethical concerns. Therapists should decline larger or more frequent gifts, including gifts of cash. Declining a small gift of low monetary value may cause unnecessary offence or precipitate a rupture in the therapeutic relationship (Australian Psychological Society, 2018).

Gift-giving from therapists to patients is not usually necessary or appropriate. But just like most boundary considerations, there may be exceptions to this rule. I once gifted a small indoor plant to a patient; the plant was not thriving in my care, and my patient took great pride in caring for and revitalising the plant. This is an example of a small gift with low monetary value. There was no expectation for the favour of a gift to be returned. Therapists who work with younger patients or families often provide small gifts, such as chocolate or confectionary, at times such as Christmas.

Boundary violations

A boundary violation represents a serious breach of the therapist's professional and ethical obligations. These actions are ethically and professionally unsound. Boundary violations are harmful and exploitative of patients, while representing some form of secondary gain for the therapist (Barnett et al., 2014).

Some actions are easily recognised as boundary violations. For example, therapists must never engage in any type of sexual activity with patients. This represents a clear boundary violation. Rules around sexual activity and intimate relationships are clearly stipulated in all professional codes of conduct and are typically also covered by legislation related to provision of health services.

Boundary violations typically begin as boundary crossings. Consistent or frequent boundary crossings can be a precursor to boundary violations. This is sometimes referred to as a "slippery slope". Left unchecked, actions or behaviours that may initially seem relatively benign or innocuous progress to being problematic, unethical, unprofessional, and, in some cases, illegal.

Therapeutic relationships

Therapists have an important role in the lives of patients. However, it is important to remember that therapists represent only one part of their patient's lives. Over-involvement in a patient's life or over-investment in the patient's therapy can have a deleterious effect on the therapeutic relationship. This can also be a key precipitant to boundary crossings and, in more serious instances, boundary violations.

> *"Don't forget that it's just a job – our patients cope*
> *for the other 167 hours in the week."*

Specifically, boundaries around therapeutic relationships are often considered in terms of *multiple relationships* and *dual roles*. These interrelated terms are used to describe crossover between therapists' professional and personal relationships. Multiple relationships and dual roles may be unavoidable, or not necessary to avoid. However, they must always be carefully managed.

> *"Try not to be over-responsible for your clients.*
> *They are responsible for their own progress."*

Multiple relationships

Multiple relationships occur when a therapist engages in additional relationships with a patient outside of the established therapeutic relationship. This may also include contact or engagement with another significant person from the patient's life, such as a family member or friend. Multiple relationships may occur in social, professional, or business settings (Barnett et al., 2014).

Not all multiple relationships can or should be avoided. Key to the appropriateness of a multiple relationship is thorough consideration and assessment of the risk of potential harm to the patient and the therapeutic relationship. Just like all decision-making around boundaries and competence in therapy, decisions should be regularly reviewed. The viability and appropriateness of the therapeutic relationship may change over time and as circumstances change. For example, a situation in which the children of the therapist and patient attend the same school can be effectively managed but must be reconsidered in the instance of the children forming a friendship that is likely to lead to shared social outings.

Conversely, the best interests of a patient may actually be met allowing a multiple relationship to proceed. For example, patients in rural areas are typically limited in choice of therapist due to fewer professionals working in remote settings. Denying a patient therapeutic intervention may be deemed more harmful that managing a multiple relationship.

Dual roles

Dual roles are conceptually similar to multiple relationships and may be governed by the same decision-making principles. Typically, however, dual roles refer to holding multiple formal roles associated with the care of the patient; for example, providing both assessment and therapy to a patient. This relatively common dual role can be managed.

Other dual roles are inappropriate and should be avoided. For example, many therapists also work in academic or teaching settings. Providing tuition or research supervision to a patient represents an inappropriate dual role that should be avoided. A therapist receiving professional amenities – such as hairdressing, financial advice, or trade or building services – also represents inappropriate dual roles that may be considered a boundary violation.

Managing multiple relationships and dual roles

In most instances, multiple relationships and dual roles can be effectively managed. Key to this is clear decision-making and awareness of ethical and professional obligations. A healthy dose of common sense is also essential. Therapists should think about how they might like to be treated in instances where a professional and personal association exists with their own therapist.

The management of multiple relationships and dual roles is a central consideration in all training courses. It represents a well-researched topic, with a plethora of resources and decision-making information available for therapists to consult.

The same decision-making applicable to general ethical dilemmas can be applied to dilemmas related to multiple relationships and dual roles (see Chapter 9). Further practical considerations and strategies include:

- Remember that as a therapist, you are a person, too. Being a therapist does not preclude any individual from the need for social affiliation or engaging in leisure activities. However, consideration needs to be given to balance both personal needs and professional responsibility.

- Allow patients to take the lead regarding communication and contact during unexpected social encounters, such as at the supermarket or at a party. Doing this lets the therapist gauge the patient's expectations and wishes for contact, which can then be reciprocated. This may include no acknowledgement or contact.
- When appropriate, pre-emptively discuss these issues with the patient. For example, a therapist who anticipates seeing a patient in a shared social setting such as the local supermarket, or a community event such as a sporting match, may ask for their preference on how to manage such meetings.

Professional relationships

Therapists interact with a variety of professionals in the course of providing treatment to patients. Dependent on work context and patient population, these may include: other therapists, referrers (such as family doctors), teachers, administrative staff (internal and external to the therapist's practice or workplace), case managers, and lawyers or other legal professionals.

Therapists working on multidisciplinary teams typically work closely and collaboratively with other professionals, such as medical doctors and other allied health professionals. Therapists working in private practice or clinic settings may be less accustomed to interactions with other professionals.

Managing professional relationships

In the same way that therapists practise in an ethical and professional manner with patients, it is imperative to maintain professional standards in any interaction with professionals outside of one's own field.

When receiving correspondence or enquiries from other professionals, therapists should ensure professional and courteous behaviour while also ensuring adherence to ethical obligations regarding confidentiality, freedom of information, and responding appropriately to subpoenas and other requests for patient files of information. For instance, it is imperative to check that the patient has given consent for their information to be released or communicated to another professional.

Therapists unsure of their obligations or responsibilities around communication with other professionals should consult the relevant professional code of ethics or seek advice in the form of supervision or from professional bodies' advisory services. If in doubt, therapists should be mindful of providing time and space to make an appropriate decision. In these instances, provide a brief reply giving a time frame by which a response will be provide, during which time the therapist can seek supervision or advice. Being rushed and feeling compelled to provide an immediate response is often a precipitant to poor decision-making.

The professional obligations and work parameters of other professionals will likely differ from that of therapists. For example, therapists do not typically work with individual members of the same family; however, this is normal practice for family doctors and some other professionals. Therapists must be careful to not project assumptions of their own professional standards or usual practices onto other professionals. Outside of instances of criminal or illegal behaviour, it is not appropriate to comment on aspects of the behaviour of another professional. This includes matters related to other professionals' incomes, or financial arrangements such as fee schedules or billing practices. Also remember that any comments made in an online community or group chat are not assured of remaining private; "closed groups" can be infiltrated, information assumed to be shared in confidence may be shared beyond the group members via screenshots or other methods.

"Always be professional even if a colleague is not!"

Self-disclosure

Self-disclosure in the context of therapy refers to a therapist making revelations about aspects of their personal life to patients. When employed with discretion and appropriate foresight, self-disclosure can be a useful therapeutic tool. It may be particularly useful in building rapport, or normalising a patient's concerns. Self-disclosure may comprise personal information, demographic details such as age, anecdotes, experiences, or personal perspectives or views.

To this end, there is a distinction between transparency and self-disclosure. A therapist can demonstrate warmth, effusiveness, and openness without disclosing detailed information about their personal life. Further, even without verbal self-disclosure, indications of a therapist's personality and life abound – clothing, grooming, speech, the furnishing of a consulting room and the books on the shelves within it. A therapist need not hide themselves from a patient, but must be mindful of unnecessarily disclosing information that may be counterproductive to therapy (Yalom, 2009).

Therapists who frequently utilise self-disclosure (or those who often feel the urge to self-disclose), whether as a general strategy or with specific patients, are encouraged to consider their own experiences of countertransference (see Chapter 8). The introspection necessary to this lends itself well to discussion in supervision or personal therapy (see Chapter 10).

Self-disclosure should be used with caution. Key considerations around self-disclosure include: being aware of the beneficiary of self-disclosure, confidentiality, being mindful of inviting further speculation, discussing politics and current events, and avoiding disclosures about third parties, including children.

The patient – not the therapist – should always be the beneficiary of self-disclosure

Self-disclosure must always be for the benefit of the patient, not the therapist. The therapist's sharing of an anecdote, experience, or any kind of personal information should be done only when in the interests of the patient. This may be to build rapport, normalise an experience or behaviour, or explain or demonstrate a psychological concept.

Self-disclosure is never an opportunity for the therapist to talk about their own problems or concerns, boast about their own achievements, or talk socially about other people.

The information disclosed should be expressed in a brief and direct manner. Consider sharing only a brief overview of the information; details (such as place, time, and other people involved) are not usually necessary to share to illustrate a point. Superfluous details typically distract from the intended purpose of the self-disclosure.

Prior to any form of self-disclosure, the therapist should reflect about the purpose and suitability of the self-disclosure.

The following questions may help:

- Who is benefitting from this self-disclosure?
- Is this disclosure going to benefit my patient?
- Is this self-disclosure motivated by my own needs? This might include a therapist's own need to share information, need for praise from the patient, or impulse to boast about themselves and their own experiences.
- Could this self-disclosure cause any rift or rupture in the therapeutic relationship?

Confidentiality

Patients are not bound to the same ethical or professional obligations as therapists around confidentiality. Any discussion in the context of therapy could be repeated to others. Therapists can and should expect that anything shared with patients may be shared with other people outside of the consulting room.

Following self-disclosure, the therapist has no control over how their personal information is used or further communicated. Like all second-hand information, the self-disclosure could be misconstrued or misinterpreted. Therapists should be mindful of this before disclosing any personal information or sharing any personal experiences.

Anticipating follow-up questions or speculation

Self-disclosure may invite reciprocity. It is social etiquette to follow up information with further questions; however, reciprocity is characteristic of personal rather than therapeutic relationships. This can be problematic for therapists, with regard to maintaining boundaries and working in a manner that is both ethically and professionally sound.

Therapists' revelations of personal information could lead to further queries or speculation. Sometimes, a little information can create an appetite for more. The therapist needs to be aware of this when considering self-disclosure. Pre-emptively deciding on a response to further queries can be helpful in maintaining boundaries.

Expectations of reciprocity or instances of speculation may be difficult or problematic for the therapist. This can be particularly pertinent in the context of changing personal circumstances, such as those within one's family or relationships. For example, a therapist experiencing relationship difficulties or the breakdown of a relationship may be upset by a patient's well-intentioned queries about the partner or spouse whom the therapist has previously spoken about. It would not be appropriate for the therapist to discuss their relationship problems with a patient; however, difficulty can arise when some precedent for discussing relationships has already been set by the therapist. This speaks to the slippery nature of professional boundaries and encourages therapists to carefully consider sharing personal information. Keep in mind that just like patients, therapists also invariably experience change in their personal lives and circumstances (Adams, 2024).

A further example is a therapist sharing an anecdote about their own childhood or schooling experiences. This may lead to specific questions about the therapist's background, such as the geographical area in which they were raised or where they attended school. In sharing any of this information, consider whether these details are relevant to therapy, or the patient and their therapeutic goals. General information is usually appropriate (such as major city or state), specific details such as a particular school or suburb is not typically necessary.

Discussing politics, religion, and current events

Most people – including therapists – live in a social vacuum in which their political and philosophical views are reinforced by media and other content with which they engage. Friends and family often provide an echo chamber of consistent thoughts and opinions. Therapists should be mindful of assuming that others will share views common to their own social group. This could unnecessarily cause a rupture in the therapeutic relationship.

A therapist should never assume a patient will share their political views or have consistent opinions on topical issues. A therapist expressing an overt opinion on political matters or commenting on world events is neither necessary nor appropriate. Therapy is not a soapbox for political views and should never be used to recruit a patient to a social movement or philosophy.

Some therapists openly share their religious or spiritual affiliation; this is often appropriate if a patient is seeking to engage with a therapist whose belief system is consistent with their own.

A therapist feeling reservation or discomfort about working with patients with whom they hold disparate political and social views should explore their concerns in supervision or their own personal therapy. Of course, it is not incumbent on every therapist to work with every patient; however, it is worthwhile to explore the reasons for reluctance or ambivalence around working with specific patients or groups of patients.

Disclosures about other people, including children

Never disclose information about another person who has not or cannot give consent to having their information shared. This includes but is not limited to children (both the therapist's own children or others they may know).

The benefits derived from self-disclosure come from the take-home message or concept being demonstrated from an anecdote or relaying of personal information. This is not usually dependent on the inclusion of specific names, ages of people, or locations. When therapeutically appropriate to refer to other people, use pronouns (he, she, they) rather than names, and general terms (at the park, at the store) rather than specific locations or store names.

Keep the focus on the patient by keeping the focus off other people.

**

My own experiences of self-disclosure relate not only to being a therapist, but also in being a writer. As a writer, I share some aspects of my personal life. This is usually in the context of providing background information or context for a specific topic. Indeed, throughout this text there are personal anecdotes and references to my professional experiences.

The personal information typically includes innocuous facts (hobbies, favourite books, conversations and observations, countries travelled to). Sparingly, I include aspects of my life that are more significant or personal, such as broad information related to relationships, my experiences of parenting, and professional and personal opinions on topical issues and current events (Denny, 2023, 2024, 2025). I am mindful to never share information about people whose permission has not been obtained. Information that may make a third party identifiable is anonymised or omitted. Like most writers, I receive both positive and negative feedback; my policy is to never respond to hostile communication (whether virtual or delivered via post) and to provide a polite but brief response to other personal correspondence. I decline requests for further information and have made a conscious decision to not speak about details of my personal life through mediums such as podcasts or other interviews.

I am guarded with personal information and usually write only of relational themes and broad experiences. However, there are implicit revelations in any of these disclosures. Certainly, some readers (often erroneously) assume to know much about me based on the scant information available in the public domain; I know this through both written and verbal comments. While others' opinions or perceptions cannot be controlled, I am assured that the narrative remains mine – I reveal aspects of my "public self" sparingly, nothing of importance about my "private self", and absolutely nothing of my "secret self".

This concept of parts of the self is represented by the Johari Window (Luft & Ingham, 1955) (see Figure 5.1). Acknowledging that each person

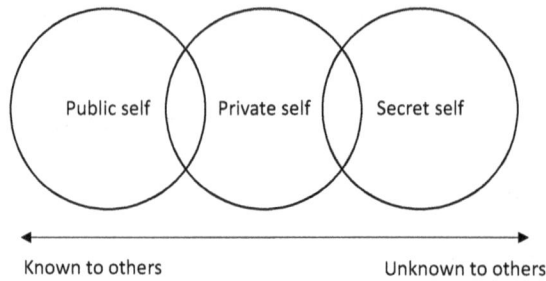

Figure 5.1 Public, private, and secret aspects of the self.

has different parts of the self that to varying degrees can be displayed or inhibited can assist when thinking about self-disclosure and appropriate sharing of personal information during therapeutic relationships.

Well-known therapists such as Irvin Yalom (2017) and Viktor Frankl (1963) have written extensively about their respective professional and personal lives and the juxtaposition between the two. More recently, Lori Gottlieb's (2022) semi-autobiographical book, *Maybe You Should Talk to Someone*, demonstrates the blending of professional and personal anecdotes. Gottlieb has further established a public brand through contributing to media outlets and sharing personal and professional information via social media.

Trainee and early-career therapists should exercise caution in following the lead of these examples of self-disclosure. Yalom and Gottlieb are experienced therapists; years of training and clinical work have no doubt contributed to their knowledge and acumen of managing their public profiles. Such high-profile professionals typically also have editors, managers, or marketing agencies who assist with decisions regarding public information and avenues for disseminating information. It is noteworthy that Yalom began his writing career relatively late in his professional career as a psychiatrist; his self-revelatory writing commenced after establishing himself as a researcher and academic author. In his later works, Yalom reflected on his "open book" philosophy in sharing his personal and professional insight, expressing concern that he may have been assumptive or cavalier at times (Yalom & Yalom, 2024).

Separate to therapists such as Yalom and Gottlieb, the late Viktor Frankl had an extraordinary story to tell; his harrowing experiences in concentration camps during World War II were integral to his world-view and the development and pioneering of a therapeutic modality called logotherapy (Frankl, 1963). Sharing his experiences was one way to demonstrate his personal and professional investment and belief in logotherapy.

Perhaps best known for his quote about the gap between stimuli and response, Frankl's personal story spoke to his belief in the power of the mind during times of adversity. (Similar to CBT in identifying and modifying thoughts, logotherapy espouses adversity as an opportunity to search for meaning in life.)

Managing self-disclosure

Beginner therapists are often concerned that patients will ask personal questions. In truth, however, few patients are interested in the personal lives of their therapist. For most patients, the hour or so spent in therapy is a rare opportunity to talk about themselves and their concerns. Therapy is by necessity an egocentric exercise.

For some patients, learning about their therapist's life is a little like seeing the man behind the screen of *The Wizard of Oz*; "real life" detail can disrupt the process and impact the patient's focus on themselves and their therapeutic goals. For this reason, many patients will resist any self-disclosure from a therapist (Yalom, 2009).

While most patients are suitably disinterested in their therapist's life, some patients do express curiosity or ask personal questions. This may be well-intentioned, with the patient assuming that the therapeutic relationship is similar to a friendship in which conversations and queries are reciprocated. Patients may say something such as, "I haven't even asked about how you are!", or "Enough about me . . . tell me about you". Deflecting questions or putting the focus on the therapist rather than themselves may represent a therapy-interfering behaviour. Whether conscious or unconscious on behalf of the patient, therapists must be mindful of therapy-interfering behaviours that can impact the pace and progress of therapy.

These are opportunities to educate the patient about therapy, rather than an invitation to share personal information. Remember, patients do not necessarily know "how to do" therapy; it is incumbent upon the therapist to share knowledge about the process of therapy, including the role of both therapist and patient, and the inherent focus on the patient rather than the therapist.

A small subset of patients may be motivated to ask personal questions for less auspicious reasons. This will depend on factors such as the patient population and presenting problems. Therapists should always be mindful of their own safety when working with patients who may present a risk for stalking or harassment. Therapists working with patients with personality disorders or forensic backgrounds need to be especially cognisant of the type and amount of self-disclosure. This does not necessarily mean that no information should be shared; rather, the therapist needs to be sophisticated in considering issues of transference and countertransference (Sperry, 2016).

It may be useful to have a "script" or list of personal details deemed appropriate to share with patients. This will comprise different information and detail for each therapist and each patient-therapist dyad. For example, it may be suitable to tell a patient that you have children, but it is generally unnecessary and inappropriate to detail the children's names, ages, or school they attend.

Be mindful of items such as personal photographs or children's drawings that may elicit queries or comments from patients. Be pre-emptively sensitive to your patients and their needs around these items; for example, photographs or other indications of a therapist's home life or children may cause unnecessary distress for perinatal patients or those experiencing fertility problems.

A therapist should never feel pressured to disclose personal information. A useful therapeutic strategy in this instance is to re-direct the conversation. This re-direction should be in a manner that is clear but non-shaming. For example, "Let's keep the focus on you", or "I'm interested to hear more about you". Remind the patient of the parameters of the therapeutic relationship and the usefulness of keeping focus on the patient and their experiences. A statement such as "I notice that our conversations keep drifting back to me . . ." may be useful to initiate a discussion about the patient's tendency to ask personal questions of the therapist.

Online behaviour

The Internet and the increasingly ubiquitous use of technology for a wide variety of tasks has, in many respects, outpaced therapy. Traditionally, therapy was a profession in which the anonymity and privacy of the therapist was not only respected but expected.

Most current trainee and early-career therapists will be "digital natives", meaning the Internet preceded their birth. These therapists were likely raised with technology and are, in comparison to previous generations of therapists, proficient in its use. Their digital footprint was likely established by others in their life, such as parents.

Trainee and early-career therapists may also have an online presence that was established prior to their commencing of training or professional work as a therapist. The content or representation may not be consistent with the therapist's professional reputation, or it may contain information that the therapist does not wish to share with people associated with their professional role, such as referrers, colleagues, or patients. Online parasocial relationships are best avoided.

Social media use and social media policy

Social media is an increasingly common advertising and marketing tool among therapists, clinics, and group therapy practices. This is an effective and often cost-efficient way to obtain referrals. Some therapists build a professional profile through social media platforms. When engaging in social media, therapists should be mindful of the potential for crossover between personal and professional information, including sharing information about locations, social or leisure activities, colleagues, and friends or family members. Information about patients should never be shared, even if anonymised.

Social media is not a place to seek specific advice or guidance on an ethical dilemma or professional quandary. It is never a replacement for supervision or professional development activities.

Online groups such as those on Facebook or other social media channels are popular among therapists. These present a good opportunity for networking and connection in a profession that can, by its very nature, be isolating. Such groups can be ideal for advertising services, discovering professional development opportunities, keeping up to date with current professional news and events, and connecting with other like-minded therapists. However, these platforms should never be used to seek specific advice or guidance on an ethical dilemma or professional quandary, or to obtain advice about specific patients and their presentations. It is never a replacement for supervision. Introspection on behalf of the therapist is helpful here; consider how you might feel as a patient if your therapist's main source of advice was from an online forum.

Settings of these groups are invariably set to "private", but this provides little assurance or guarantee that information will not be shared outside of the group. Information related to specific patients or patient presentations should never be shared in online groups or in other online forums. This includes but is not limited to patients' names, ages, schools or workplaces, or specific location. If seeking an onward referral, it is sufficient to state the patient's general age, presentation, and location. For example, "Adolescent, presentation of anxiety and school refusal, central Sydney". This provides enough initial information without inadvertently identifying the patient.

Professional codes of conduct are increasingly including guidelines around use of technology and social media. In conjunction with these, therapists should refer back to general information contained in ethical guidelines and professional codes of conduct. Core principles (such as confidentiality, professional boundaries, beneficence, and propriety) remain key for all professional conduct, whether virtual or in person.

A "social media policy" may be included as part of the informed consent process. This should be updated regularly to reflect changes in the social media landscape. Therapists have a responsibility to manage parasocial relationships that can arise from social media and social networking sites.

Being pre-emptively declarative about expectations around social media is likely to save both the therapist and patient from any potential difficulties that may arise. The policy may stipulate agreement around issues such as:[1]

- "Friending"
  - Therapists should decline any friend requests on social networking sites from current or former patients.
  - Some therapists opt to have no social networking presence or profile. This is one way to avoid potential interactions with patients; however, alternatives exist such as setting clear boundaries around use, opting for high privacy settings, and using an assumed or alternative name. Be mindful, however, that none of these measures can provide a complete guarantee of privacy or anonymity.
- "Fanning" or "following"
  - Online "fanning" or "following" is typically more passive than "friending", as a patient is able to "fan" or "follow" a therapist's professional social networking page without the therapist's explicit approval or agreement.
  - The therapist should consider whether this is appropriate for their therapy practice, including potential consequences of the dual relationship brought about by "fanning" or "following".
- Online interactions
  - Therapists should refrain from online interactions with patients.
  - Declining friendship requests and not reciprocating "fanning" or "following" is one way to minimise further instances of online interaction.
- Online searches
  - Therapists should never conduct online searches of their patients.
- Business review sites
  - Therapists should never solicit endorsements or testimonials from patients.

- Therapists should not respond to online endorsements, reviews, or testimonials.
- In some countries, such as Australia, testimonials for therapy services are explicitly banned by the national regulatory body.
- Electronic messages, including email, text messaging, and chat services
  - Typically, therapists use these instant messaging services for administrative tasks, such as appointment scheduling and invoicing.
  - Guidelines may be developed to ensure shared expectations around the use of these services for communication from patients, such as to receive homework tasks or other documents.
  - Patients should be reminded that any electronic communication, such as that received via email or text message, is retained as part of their patient file.
  - Email and instant messaging do not constitute a crisis service. Therapists may consider noting this as part of informed consent paperwork or also providing this information in an email signature.

Summary

- In the context of therapy and therapeutic relationships, boundaries refer to the professional behaviour of a therapist, particularly in relation to therapeutic relationships with patients.
- Boundaries are typically thought of in relation to direct patient work. Boundaries also extend to professional behaviour in relation to third parties and other professionals with whom the therapist may interact or communicate.
- Boundaries exist on a spectrum. Boundaries are often not black-and-white, and as such the distinction between boundary crossings and boundary violations can be difficult to discern.
- A boundary crossing, also referred to as a boundary transgression, refers to a clinically appropriate course of action that is deemed appropriate by both the therapist and the patient.
- A boundary violation refers to behaviours that contravene professional standards. These are typically harmful and may be exploitative of the patient.
- Dual roles and multiple relationships that cannot be avoided must be carefully managed in order to ensure the therapist continues to practise in a manner that provides therapeutic benefit to the patient and does not breach any professional or ethical obligation.

- Overlap often occurs between therapeutic relationships and other roles, such as social groups, membership of an organisation, or affiliation with a school or similar organisation. Mutual acquaintances are also likely. These may be more common in rural or remote areas, but they can impact all therapeutic relationships regardless of location.
- Self-disclosure in therapy refers to the revelations about the therapist's personal information or experiences.
- Considerations for self-disclosure include confidentiality, caution around fuelling speculation about the therapist or inviting further queries, and being mindful of information pertaining to third parties, including children and others who have not consented to their information being shared.
- Self-disclosure must always be in the interest of the patient, rather than to satisfy an unmet need of the therapist.
- A therapist's online presence and behaviour has implications for their professional standing and may also impact therapeutic relationships and professional boundaries. Therapists should be aware of their online presence and have clear expectations and guidelines around online interaction with patients.
- Parasocial relationships between therapists and relationship are best avoided. This includes interactions via social media and other online platforms.

Note

1   Adapted from Kolmes (2020) March 26, 2025, 3:12:00 PM

Reference list

Adams, M. (2024). *The myth of the untroubled therapist* (2nd ed.). Routledge.

Australian Psychological Society. (2018). The giving and taking of gifts. *InPsych*, 40(6).

Barnett, J. E., Zimmerman, J., & Walfish, S. (2014). *The ethics of private practice: A practical guide for mental health clinicians*. Oxford University Press.

Denny, B. (2023, November 6). How shame influences the decisions we make, and compounds the harm we do to others. *ABC Religion & Ethics*. https://www.abc.net.au/religion/shame-regret-and-the-reasons-for-the-decisions-we-make/103070984

Denny, B. (2024, September 8). It's a nice idea, but more therapy won't fix our growing mental health crisis. *The Age*.

Denny, B. (2025). *Talk to me: Lessons from patients and their therapist.* Routledge.

Frankl, V. E. (1963). *Man's search for meaning.* Washington Square Press.

Gabbard, G. O. (2005). *Psychodynamic psychiatry in clinical practice* (4th ed.). American Psychiatric Publications.

Gottlieb, L. (2022). *Maybe you should talk to someone: A therapist, her therapist, and our lives revealed.* Scribe Publications.

Kolmes, K. (2020). *My private practice social media policy.* https://drkkolmes.com/docs/socmed.pdf

Luft, J., & Ingham, H. (1955). The Johari window, a graphic model of interpersonal awareness. In *Proceedings of the western training laboratory in group development.* UCLA.

McNulty, N., Ogden, J., & Warren, F. (2013). "Neutralizing the patient": Therapists' accounts of sexual boundary violations. *Clinical Psychology & Psychotherapy, 20*(3), 189–198. https://doi.org/10.1002/cpp.799

McWilliams, N. (1999). *Psychoanalytical case formulation.* Guilford Press.

Sperry, L. (2016). *Handbook of diagnosis and treatment of DSM-5 personality disorders: Assessment, case conceptualization, and treatment* (3rd ed.). Routledge.

Yalom, I. D. (2009). *The gift of therapy: Reflections on being a therapist.* Harper Perennial.

Yalom, I. D. (2017). *Becoming myself: A psychiatrist's memoir.* Scribe Publications.

Yalom, I. D., & Yalom, B. (2024). *Hour of the heart: Connecting in the here and now.* Scribe Publications.

Therapist competence and confidence 6

Therapists are both ethically and professionally obliged to be competent in delivering services and treatment. The balance between competence (actual capacity) and confidence (self-assessment of capacity) presents challenges for many therapists, but especially those at trainee or early-career stages.

Competence

Competence refers to the capacity of a therapist to effectively and efficiently complete the tasks required of their role. This encompasses several core areas for therapists, including knowledge, clinical skills, and ethical values and professional behaviours. Specific competencies related to therapy include communication, and clinical reasoning and judgement.

A competent therapist has the ability to integrate knowledge and skills in order to provide effective care to patients. They practice in a manner that is ethically and professionally sound, ensuring their knowledge and skills are up to date and reflective of current professional expectations and standards. A competent therapist has the capacity for independent work and autonomous decision-making, while seeking supervision and guidance as required.

> *"There's no such thing as a dumb question,*
> *so please don't be scared to ask . . . this can save a*
> *lot of stress and/or heartache down the track."*

DOI: 10.4324/9781003533030-6

Competence is a dynamic and ongoing process. Scope of competence will change over time for all therapists; the level of competence expected from trainee therapists is objectively lower than that expected of those in established or senior roles. Specific roles and workplaces will also hold varied expectations regarding competence. No therapist can ever be "fully competent" in all areas of knowledge or across all types of therapies or intervention.

> *"You don't need to 'know it all', and in fact*
> *you never will. And that's okay!"*

Three main sources are relevant to therapist competence: legislation, professional codes of conduct, and workplace codes of conduct (see Figure 6.1). Therapists have a professional obligation to ensure current knowledge and understanding of each.

Legislation refers to a law or set of laws that govern a state or country. Therapists must abide by legislation, in both their professional and personal conduct. Examples of legislation relevant to therapists may include mandatory reporting (i.e., the requirement of alerting authorities when reasonable belief exists that a child or other person may be at risk of harm), freedom of information (i.e., patients' access to their records and information), and consumer law (around business dealings).

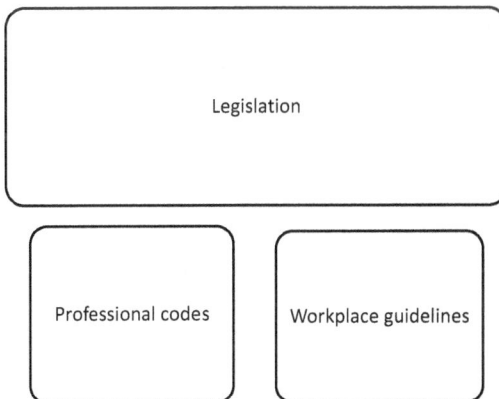

Legislation

Professional codes

Workplace guidelines

Figure 6.1 Competence is informed by three main sources: legislation, professional codes, and workplace guidelines. Legislation takes precedence in instances of conflict between the three.

Professional codes are produced by regulatory boards and licensing bodies. They may also be known as codes of conduct, codes of ethics, of professional charters. These provide documentation detailing the expectations of therapists and the parameters under which they may work. Professional codes typically have a strong focus on ethical and professional behaviour. These documents do not answer specific questions about ethical or professional dilemmas experienced by therapists but instead provide information and general rules that can be applied to specific problems. Supplementary information about specific areas and tasks of therapy may also be included, such as guidelines and rules around assessment, diagnosis, intervention, report writing, record-keeping, and working with specific populations.

Workplace guidelines are specific to places of employment. Similar to professional codes, workplace guidelines focus on professional behaviour. These guidelines may apply to a range of professions within the workplace or organisation, such as medical staff, allied health professionals, and administrative staff. The information is not usually specific to therapists.

Information presented in legislation, professional codes, and workplace guidelines may overlap. Alternatively, information across the sources may be in conflict or seem contradictory. In these instances, legislation always takes precedence over professional codes and workplace guidelines.

It is the responsibility of each individual therapist to maintain current and accurate knowledge of their professional and legal responsibilities. This will ensure that any potential discrepancies are identified as early as possible, reducing the risk of these discrepancies becoming precipitants to ethical and professional dilemmas. A lack of awareness of information stipulated in legislation, professional codes, or workplace guidelines is not considered an adequate explanation for poor professional conduct or unethical behaviour. Decision-making and additional considerations around these issues are further discussed in Chapter 9.

Measuring competence

Competence is objective and can therefore be measured against a set of standards. Many therapists will be familiar with this process from training programmes or internships; an evaluation is conducted by supervisors or other instructors, with an appraisal of the trainee's progress and standing across a range of domains. Self-assessment may also be required; this can prompt valuable discussion between trainee and their supervisors. It is also especially useful to initiate the practice of self-supervision (see Chapter 10).

*"Adopt a beginner's mind, always, not just in
the early stages of becoming a therapist. Then we
are as open as we can possibly be to all the potential
ways of viewing or understanding our
patient's experience."*

The purpose of evaluation – whether with a supervisor or via self-reflection – is to obtain an indication of current standing with a view to identifying areas for improvement. This can then inform a professional development plan designed to increase competence as necessary. To this end, "success" in evaluation of competence need not mean excelling or gaining full marks in all areas. Instead, the focus is on identifying strengths and areas for improvement.

Areas of competence typically included in codes of conduct or guidelines for professional practice encompass:

• Knowledge
• Communication
• Ethical and professional practice
• Self-reflection, self-care
• Assessment
• Intervention

Competence vs confidence

Four stages of competence (see Figure 6.2) apply to the learning of any skill and mastery of a practice, including therapy. Progression through the four stages is typically sequential; however, individual differences may exist. While the model of competence and confidence is often discussed in terms of trainee therapists, it also applies to therapists at later career stages who may be commencing a new role or learning a new skill set, such as that related to a new therapeutic modality. Given that the profession of therapy requires lifelong learning to maintain competence, all therapists will at times find themselves at varying points of the four stages of competence. An ability to identify the stage of competence assists in ensuring the therapist practises within the scope of their current competence and ability.

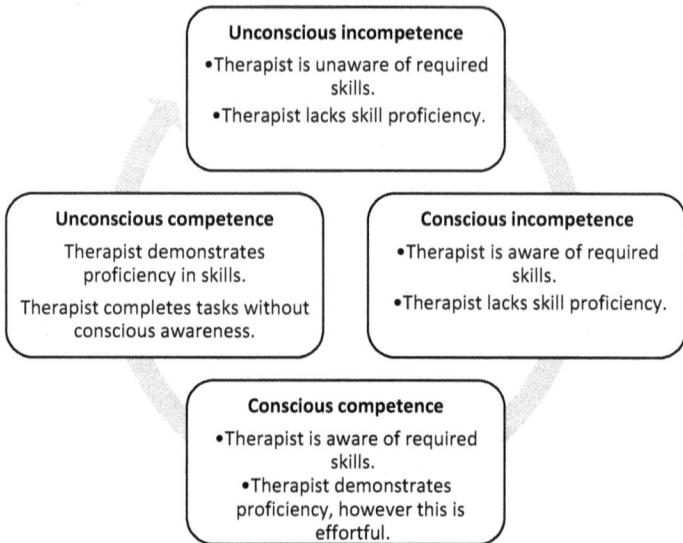

Figure 6.2 Four stages of competence for therapists.

Stage 1 – Unconscious incompetence

"Unconsciously incompetent" best describes most therapists at the commencement of training. That is, beginner therapists are aware of the massive task of learning ahead of them, but they are unaware of the specific skills required and their own lack of proficiency around these skills.

"Just get started, you will learn along the way."

Stage 2 – Conscious incompetence

As training progresses, therapists gain awareness of the specific skills and tasks required to establish and maintain a competent level of practice. This stage of "conscious incompetence" may be characterised by feelings of overwhelm, as the therapist realises the extent of the learning and work ahead.

"You know more than you think you do."

Stage 3 – Conscious competence

The therapist has acquired necessary skills and demonstrates proficiency in many aspects of the knowledge and application of therapy. However, applying these skills and delivering therapeutic treatment takes concerted effort. At this stage, the therapist is acutely aware of both their level of competence and areas that require further learning or improvement.

"You have to learn to sit with a certain level of discomfort."

Stage 4 – Unconscious competence

The therapist delivers treatment in a confident manner and without conscious concerns about their skills. Therapists at this stage have both the confidence and competence required to instruct other therapists and are well-placed to work in supervisory or teaching roles.

"It's a long journey, and you're only at the beginning.
Know that with each passing year your confidence and
competence will grow. Even as you recognise over time you
know less and less about the human condition. Still, you're
willing to give helping another person a go."

"The 'real' learning really does begin after you graduate!
And adding to that, you will never stop learning . . ."

Imposter syndrome

Therapists are generally prone to self-examination. In many ways this is a useful skill, but at times this introspection, combined with a tendency towards perfectionistic thinking, can lead therapists to ponder about their own standing, particularly in comparison to other therapists. This phenomenon of comparing the self to others and having a response of feeling that one is fraudulent and does not belong has become known as imposter syndrome. Imposter syndrome can encompass self-doubt, a lack of belonging, intellectual inferiority, and feeling undeserving of success or achievement.

Like many therapists, I have experienced (and continue to experience) imposter syndrome. These thoughts were especially prevalent at the beginning of my professional training. Prior to commencing postgraduate training in a clinical psychology programme, I took an overseas trip for the long summer break. My enjoyment of the trip was tinged with increasing anxiety about commencing professional training. The anticipated workload and steep learning were the initial focus of my concerns. I felt overwhelmed at the prospect of combining course work, professional placements, and a large research thesis. But as the trip progressed, my worries were increasingly dominated by thoughts of deservedness of having obtained a place in a highly sought-after training course. I convinced myself that the letter of offer from the University (delivered via post in those pre-Internet days) was a result of an administrative error. Surely, I reasoned internally, the letter had been incorrectly addressed and never intended for me. It was all an administration blunder. The fraudulence of my position in the course would soon be discovered, and I would be unceremoniously dumped from the programme before even having had a chance to commence it. I played down congratulations and platitudes from my travel companions about being accepted into the training programme, embarrassed at the prospective notion of having to explain in the future that my admission had been an error.

My experience of imposter syndrome continued to the first class of our first semester. I assumed the other 14 trainee therapists in the cohort to be naturally assured and infinitely more skilled. While I was now assured of my place in the programme (there had been no retraction correspondence in the letter box upon my arrival home from overseas), my imposter syndrome changed shape and presented itself in a different way: I automatically relegated myself to the bottom of the academic pile. I was convinced the others were more competent and confident. Sooner or later, I thought, my ineptitude would be apparent to all.

I now recognise my experience of imposter syndrome to be a type of defence mechanism. I convinced myself of the worst-case scenario in an unconscious effort to better cope with the potential disappointment of not proceeding with the training course or performing badly within it.

"We don't need to be perfect."

Like many psychology or therapy-speak terms, language around the phenomenon of imposter syndrome is now used beyond its original definition.

Imposter syndrome is not now, nor ever has been, a clinical diagnosis. It is not recognised in the *Diagnostic and Statistical Manual of Mental Disorders* (DSM; American Psychiatric Association, 2013) or other diagnostic texts.

The phenomenon was first formally identified and investigated in the late 1970s, with research focused on the self-doubt commonly experienced by high-achieving women employed in prestigious roles (Clance & Imes, 1978). Despite being qualified (and, in some cases, overqualified) for the roles in which they were employed, the women reported feelings of imposition, inferiority, lack of confidence, and concerns around deservedness. The researchers also noted observations about gender differences, with men thought to experience less imposter syndrome than women, even in instances of objectively inferior qualifications or professional experience.

Factors theorised as likely contributors to the imposter phenomenon included a tendency to attribute success to an external rather than internal source (i.e., luck or good fortune over hard work), traits of perfectionism that had likely developed during childhood or early family experiences, doubts about one's own intelligence or academic abilities, and the tendency to focus on negative rather than positive feedback (Clance & Imes, 1978).

"It's okay to not know everything."

The contexts in which therapists train and work provide an ideal breeding ground for imposter syndrome. Trainee and early-career therapists often report feelings of self-doubt and overwhelm, thoughts of incompetence, and worries about inferiority. This is often exacerbated by comparison to peers and assumptions about the competence and confidence of others.

The experience of feeling like an imposter can be distressing. It is associated with compassionate fatigue and can also precipitate burnout (Clark et al., 2022; Türkel et al., 2025). In an effort to avoid distress, therapists may naturally want to push away or deny these thoughts. Reassurance from friends or colleagues may be sought; on some level the therapist may be hoping their thoughts of imposition will be countered by encouragement or positivity, or elicit empathy in the form of stories about similar experiences.

Rather than automatically seeking to push away or provide an explanation or justification for such thoughts, benefit can arise from instead acknowledging and leaning into them. Tapping into these thoughts and feelings encourages useful self-reflection and promotes awareness and insight about strengths and areas for improvement. This can be key for personal development, and also professional development in terms of directions for further training and skill development. Personal therapy and professional supervision have also been posited as useful to resolving the self-doubt and emotional dysregulation common to the imposter phenomenon (DeCandia Vitoria, 2021).

"Allow yourself to make mistakes and try new things."

Rather than deny or minimise thoughts of imposition, consider the *meaning* and *origins* of the experience of imposter phenomenon. The following prompt may be useful to encourage self-reflection, or to discuss the experience of imposter phenomenon in supervision or with colleagues:

1. Evaluate your skill level and level of experience:
    - Are your thoughts about being an imposter founded?
    - Is unfair comparison being made with other therapists, particularly those who have more experience or training with specific patient populations or presenting problems?
2. Consider your scope of practice:
    - You are not expected to be competent in all aspects of therapy or to practise all therapeutic modalities or interventions.
    - Be aware of your strengths and areas for improvement.
    - Resist pressure (from referrers, clients, employers) to accept referrals that do not fit within your scope of practice.
3. Consider what can be learned from the feelings of imposition:
    - What training or professional development programmes could I participate in to increase my understanding and skill in this experience?
4. Be a "good enough" therapist:
    - Recognise your existing skill set.
    - Be honest with yourself about your areas for improvement, but do not lose sight of your current value.
5. Engage in therapy and seek supervision:
    - It may be useful to further explore your own experience of imposter syndrome and its origins. This may be through personal therapy and, to some extent, within supervision. The origins of imposter syndrome may lie within early life experiences, trauma, or family expectations of achievement and success.
    - Also consider whether thoughts and feelings of imposter syndrome may be reflective of psychological distress, or conditions such as depression and anxiety.

Therapists at any career stage, but particularly in the early years, must give themselves permission to not know everything (Cozolino, 2004).

This is especially true of trainees and recent graduates. There can be incongruence between the internal and external selves of a therapist; while receiving praise and external validation (perhaps in the form of being looked to by friends and family for therapeutic advice), the graduate is "consciously incompetent" in knowing their strengths and limitations (see Figure 6.2). In this sense, it is useful to remember that training programmes do not contain all the answers to every query. No therapist will graduate with knowledge and skill related to all presentations and patient populations. Therapists will necessarily leave feeling that they have much still to learn. Training programmes aim to equip therapists with sufficient knowledge and skill to allow graduate therapists to enter the profession and provide safe and effective treatment to patients.

Acknowledging limitations, reinforcing strengths, focusing on achievements, and setting aspirations for future learning together represent an adaptive approach to the inevitable experience of imposter syndrome.

Selecting an area of specialty or expertise

Choosing a therapeutic modality

The term "therapeutic modality" refers to a type, style, or mode of therapy practised by a clinician. Therapies can be generally categorised into a few main groups – affective (focused on feelings), cognitive (thoughts), behavioural (actions), and systemic (relational dynamics within a unit, such as a family) (Hackney & Cormier, 2012). There are subtypes of therapies within each group. New modalities and refinements and extensions or existing modalities are also being developed.

Most trainee and graduate programmes focus on time-limited, structured treatments, such as cognitive behaviour therapy (CBT). This is a popular choice, given its application to several presenting problems and proven efficacy across a range of symptomatology (Beck & Beck, 1995). Training in acceptance and commitment therapy (ACT) is also common. Some courses include coverage of more advanced therapeutic modalities, such as psychodynamic psychotherapy, schema therapy, or dialectic behaviour therapy (DBT). The selection of therapeutic modalities covered in courses or taught by training institutions and graduate programmes are bound by curriculum requirements set by licensing boards. This may also be influenced by organisational factors, such as funding considerations and faculty research interests and expertise.

*"Expand your horizon and be open to all the
pathways your skills can take you on."*

The modalities of CBT and ACT provide an excellent foundation for trainee and early-career therapists. It is noteworthy that several other popular modalities, such as schema therapy and DBT, have their origins in CBT. This speaks to the benefit for trainee and early-career therapists in mastering common treatment approaches such as CBT, as this will give an excellent foundation upon which to build knowledge and skills of other modalities.

"Explore different modalities."

Training programmes sometimes attract criticism for failing to provide breadth of therapeutic modalities. Some trainee and early-career therapists report feeling ill-equipped for independent practice or working with patients whose presentations are novel or complex. This criticism is somewhat unfair; while all training programmes differ, the primary goal of such programmes is to provide essential introductory information that will equip therapists to enter the profession and practice in a way that is safe and ethically sound. The aim is to educate therapists about core principles of therapy; this primarily includes knowledge, ethics, and professional practice, and the application of these to clinical practice. Comprehensive coverage of these crucial areas in courses that are typically a handful of years in duration is no small feat; any trainee therapist can attest to the heavy workload and busy schedule. The importance of this foundational training should not be minimised or dismissed. The expectation is that the therapist will progress their knowledge and skill by participating in ongoing learning, such as professional development activities, further specialised training, and engaging in supervision (see Chapter 10).

*"The best thing I would say to someone straight out of training
is to make the therapy fit the person, not the other way round.
Choose the set of techniques or approaches which fit with
the individual's needs, issues and cognitive-emotional 'style'.
Eclectic customisation and flexibility are good; prescribing
treatment preferences that the patient must assimilate to is bad."*

After mastering the foundations of modalities taught in training, many mid-career therapists find themselves drawn towards wanting to learn more about a specific therapeutic modality or style. These may include extended learning about modalities that were briefly introduced during training, such as schema therapy, DBT, EMDR, psychodynamic psychotherapy, psychoanalytic psychotherapy, family therapy, group therapy, and couples or relationship therapy. Alternatively, therapists may find themselves wanting to focus on a specific patient population, such as children and adolescents, neurodivergent individuals, or patients experiencing eating disorders. Further, some therapists choose to focus their practice on assessment and diagnostic reports; this may encompass work for individuals, insurance agencies, or the forensic or court system.

Focusing on a specific population group or presentation will typically require some sort of further study, training, and specific supervision. Accreditation or certification is available for specific modalities; these are usually provided by private organisations or institutions and are usually independent of licensing boards or regulatory boards. While some therapists choose to pursue full accreditation or certification in specific modalities, extensive training in a particular modality is typically not required to apply strategies or learnings into clinical practice. For example, many therapists may use aspects of modalities such as schema therapy in their work without having completed full accreditation as a schema therapist. As always, therapists need to be mindful of their competence in specific areas and not practise beyond the scope of their training and knowledge.

"You don't need to know everything or be ready for everything, to provide people with much-needed care."

Therapists have many options for areas of work. This can be concurrently exciting and overwhelming. Similar to other professional fields, "trends" in therapy also emerge; this is noticeable in both patient queries and also the number of professional development workshops being offered in a particular field. Remember, no therapist can do it all, and no therapist needs to pivot to a new therapeutic modality at the request of patients or referrers. A particular type of therapy being popular or prevalent in the media does not necessarily mean it is the right fit for each therapist or all patients.

Therapists looking to discover their niche may be guided by the following questions:

- What interests me?
- What theory or practice feels "sparkly" for me?
- What patient population am I interested in working with?
- Which particular diagnosis or condition interests me?
- In which area of work will I feel appropriately challenged?
- What will sustain my interest over time?
- Which niche area might reliably provide a steady referral base and/or job security?

"Explore different modalities."

Practical strategies and activities may also be helpful to further explore a therapeutic modality or niche work area:

- Engage in personal therapy with a range of therapists who practise different therapeutic modalities (see Chapter 10).
- Read about different therapeutic modalities.
- Observe sessions, via recordings available online or through a resource library.
- Acknowledge that different therapeutic modalities will be appropriate for specific presentation and refer patients as appropriate. For example, a psychodynamic therapist may refer to a patient to a cognitive behaviour therapist for short-term treatment of conditions such as procrastination or insomnia.
- Establish professional acquaintance with therapists who practise various therapeutic modalities. Ask about their experiences of establishing and maintaining interest and work in their niche area. Be curious about how they came to settle on a long-term option.
- Enter a mentoring programme. These are often offered by professional organisations. Early-career therapists are matched with established therapists, promoting discussions about training options, therapeutic modalities, and career trajectory.
- Attend a variety of professional events and workshops. These provide affordable and flexible opportunities to explore modalities and niche work areas. Introductory courses may comprise workshops of one to

two days as well as webinars (live or on demand). This is an investment of time and money, but it does not lock the therapist into committing to further training. Therapists employed by organisations may receive funding for professional development and attending workshops, while self-employed therapists may be able to claim these costs as tax expenditure.

Alternatively, a good starting point for a therapist considering which therapeutic modality may be to consider what *not* to do. It is often easier to discount options rather than to decide on one. For example, areas for consideration may include specific patient populations, employment settings (such as hospitals or schools), or diagnostic conditions. Experiences from training, where therapists typically work with patients from across the lifespan and with a range of presenting problems or diagnoses, can inform a therapist's thinking about aspects of therapeutic practice they do not wish to pursue.

Some therapists, particularly those in the mid-stage of their careers, become very strongly aligned to a specific therapeutic modality. Interest and dedication to a therapeutic modality is useful, but a dogmatic approach is not. Therapists should keep an open mind about different therapeutic modalities and demonstrate respect for colleagues who may practise in a different manner or style. Disparaging a therapeutic modality outside of one's own preferred approach is never appropriate. Keeping an open mind about a variety of therapeutic modalities, even those that for whatever reason do not spark your interest or attention, helps promote the reputation of the profession of therapy as a whole. This is the most useful approach to providing optimal care and the best treatment for all patients.

Finally, remember that whatever modality or style of therapeutic work, therapy is essentially about the rapport and connection between therapist and patient (Yalom, 2009). Any therapeutic work is about best outcomes, not for the fulfilment of any therapist's ego or to prove one therapy as superior over another. Therapists should keep this in mind while balancing the nuances and intricacies of therapy work, particularly when learning advanced aspects of any therapeutic modality and intervention.

"And some final words from an intellectual great [Carl Jung]: Learn all the modalities, master all the techniques, but when you reach out to touch another human soul, just be another human soul."

Working within scope of competence, training, and experience

Scope of practice refers to the range of professional services and types of patients that a therapist can competently assess and treat (Barnett et al., 2014).

Therapists must never misrepresent themselves or their qualifications. In some countries, including Australia, terms such as "psychologist" are protected titles. This means that the title may be used only after an individual has completed a recognised course of study and is registered with a relevant licensing board. It is illegal to erroneously use a protected title to describe themselves in a personal or professional capacity. This can attract substantial penalty, including a monetary fine, possible criminal conviction, and exclusion from further training or qualifications in the professional field.

Most therapists demonstrate a good understanding of the rationale for working within one's scope and competence, training, and experience. The need to practise in a way that is both ethically and professionally sound is emphasised through undergraduate courses and postgraduate training. Sometimes, however, this does not translate clearly to the realities of clinical practice. In comparison to hypothetical vignettes presented during training, real-life scenarios are often complex and prove difficult to navigate.

Even the most conscientious therapist may lose sight of ethical and professional responsibilities when faced with stress around issues such as business considerations, workload, and financial strain. Managing professional relationships with employers, referrers, and prospective patients can also present challenges for therapists in working within their scope of competence, training, and experience. Requests for services that may sit outside the therapist's experience or expertise (such as assessment reports, diagnosis, or delivery of a specific therapeutic modality) may also lead to therapists feeling pressured to work outside of their scope of competence or experience. Two of these areas – patient selection and diagnostic considerations – are detailed here.

"Careful with your ego. You won't help everyone, and you won't get thanked by everyone."

Patient selection and referral process

Trainee and early-career therapists are understandably keen to gain experience and establish themselves in a professional standing. This represents a necessary expansion of skills and knowledge. However, expanding practice also comes with risks around stepping outside of one's area of competence, particularly around accepting referrals, building a caseload, and working with patients with diverse presentations.

Therapists do not need to have expert knowledge in every clinical presentation in order to work effectively with a range of patients. However, a minimum level of knowledge and clinical experience is required in order to work in a manner that is both professionally and ethically sound. Further, additional specific training and supervision may be needed to work with some patients and presentations.

Several sources of pressure are common precipitants to therapists working outside of their scope of competence (Barnett et al., 2014; Frankcom et al., 2016). An awareness of these can assist therapists in reflecting on their position and inform decision-making that is both ethically and professionally sound.

- Financial (needing to fill appointments to maintain financial viability of a therapy practice)
- Ego (reluctance to admit lack of proficiency or knowledge)
- Fear of disappointing referrers by declining to accept patients
- Pressure – whether implicit or explicit – from managers or practice owners to accept referrals that may not be consistent with the therapist's experience or knowledge
- Inadequate supervision and lack of consultation with colleagues regarding case load and appropriate presentations

Therapists at all career stages should be mindful of working within their scope of competence in terms of their case load (number of current patients), the patient population with whom they work, and type of presentation. This becomes clearer and easier to navigate for established therapists who likely have a reputation based on working with particular patient populations or specific presenting problems and therefore receive appropriate referrals. However, patients do not come with warning signs. Despite the best efforts of a therapist or intake service, a limited amount of information can be gleaned prior to an initial appointment. Referral information may be incomplete or inaccurate. Initial contact with a patient may not indicate the patient or their presentation to be inappropriate or beyond the scope of the therapist's skill or experience.

"It's important to know your limits and what you can/can't do. Refer on and/or get supervision and if you are not well-versed in the area. This is NOT a failing – we simply cannot know everything about everything!"

Screening of referrals through appropriate intake is imperative; however, there is no fail-safe method for intake. All therapists will at some stage find themselves sitting with a patient whose presentation or needs sit outside of their scope of competence. This might be apparent in the first session or become clear only as assessment and treatment progress. Sometimes, patients' presentations may change over time or further information may become apparent, meaning the therapist is no longer best suited to provide care.

The social psychology theory of the "sunk cost effect" is useful to remember when thinking about accepting referrals and continuing to work with patients whose presentation may sit outside your scope of competence. This theory explains the human tendency to continue an endeavour in the face of evidence that suggests discontinuation is a better option. The investment of time, money, or effort sways the individual towards less optimal decision-making. Implicated here is the desire to not be viewed by others as wasteful, incapable, or recalcitrant.

"You don't need to see all the patients. You can say no."

It may be tempting for a therapist to forge on with treatment, regardless of indications that the best course of action may be stopping treatment or providing an onward referral to another therapist. This can be due to various factors, such as a change in the patient's presentation, that puts working with the patient outside of the therapist's scope of competence. The therapist may believe that a good working relationship or therapeutic rapport can compensate for their lack of skill or knowledge in a particular area. More practical concerns may also exist, such as availability of options for onward referral. This can be particularly pertinent for therapists working in rural or remote areas, where there may be a shortage of other therapists available to accept referrals or work with patients. In this case, it is useful to communicate with the referrer regarding concerns. Individual therapists are important to patients, but a team approach helps ensure that no one clinician becomes indispensable to a patient's care.

In some instances, patients may benefit from being referred to a different service or new therapist. Another strategy is to accept the referral on a tentative basis, communicating with the patient that a decision around potential to work together for ongoing treatment will be made after completion of initial sessions.

Therapists should utilise multiple tools in decision-making about accepting patient referrals. It is the responsibility of the therapist to evaluate the suitability of a referral.

- Introspection and reflection regarding own level of competence and stage of learning.
- Professional support is available if the referral is to be accepted; for example, collegial support or supervision with therapists with expertise, or experience with a specific presenting problem or patient population.
- Follow an ethical decision-making model (see Chapter 9).
- Seek guidance and advice from colleagues and supervisors.
- Consult relevant legislation, professional codes of conduct, and workplace guidelines.

Therapists should also be mindful of pressure from prospective patients to accept referrals that sit outside of their scope of competence. Some patients are understandably anxious to secure an appointment with a therapist and may not be aware of the difference between specific therapists and their experience or expertise with specific patient populations or presenting problems. Similarly, resist pressure from referrers or other third parties (such as lawyers) to accept referrals or requests that are beyond your professional scope. Early-career therapists may feel pressure to accept a referral in order to please the referrer and build a good relationship. Remember, referrers want the best outcomes for the patient, and the best way to build a solid referral base is by providing good therapy and, by extension, good therapeutic outcomes to patients. This may mean declining some referrals. Communicate this to the referrer briefly (i.e., "I am not able to accept this referral as I currently do not work with patients within this age group and/or with this presentation"); there is no need to over-explain or provide a detailed rationale for your decision. Provide details of other therapists, if appropriate. No therapist will be competent in all areas;

this should be acknowledged rather than become a point of shame or source of disappointment.

Therapists should document their decision-making regarding referrals, particularly in instances where the referral sits outside the therapist's usual remit, or where a detailed intake phone call or initial session has been conducted. This helps solidify the process around referrals and is also useful reference documentation should any decision be queried by a registration or licensing body.

Diagnostic considerations

There is much public interest in the diagnosis of mental health conditions. This seems a result of several factors, including advocacy regarding mental illness and mental health, increased knowledge of the aetiology and treatment of mental illness, and a societal move towards individuals wanting to better understand themselves and their psyche (Denny, 2023). Diagnostic language that was once limited to use by clinicians has been adopted as common parlance.

Diagnosis may be sought for a number of reasons, including funding purposes, special consideration for study, requests for adaptations to employment conditions, or to obtain treatment including medication. Diagnosis can also be helpful in terms of aiding the search for a therapist with expertise in a specific area. Increasingly, individuals are seeking diagnosis for their own knowledge; for some, a diagnostic label for their experience is useful in terms of communicating their experience to other people, including family members and acquaintances.

Consequent to this increased understanding of mental health and mental illness is increased demand for diagnostic assessment, particularly around neurodiversity, autism spectrum disorder, and attention deficit hyperactivity disorder (ADHD). Increased public appetite and assumed understanding of diagnosis presents a somewhat vexed issue for therapists. As experts in the field of mental health and mental illness, therapists are often consulted about diagnosis. However, there is a wide variability among therapists' qualifications and diagnostic knowledge and skill. This is not always known by members of the public, who may assume all therapists hold the same qualifications and have similar diagnostic interests and capacity. For example, the role of psychiatrists and psychologists are often confused. (For the record, psychiatrists are medical doctors who have undertaken further training in mental health. Their role is often focused on diagnosis and management of psychotropic medication; however, some also provide psychotherapy.) It is therefore imperative that therapists be clear in their communication and practice around all aspects of their work, including diagnosis.

Attitudes towards diagnosis will be shaped by several factors, including the therapist's own training and therapeutic modality. Irvin Yalom (2009), the esteemed existential psychotherapist, adopts a relational approach to diagnosis, in that he discourages diagnosis outside of instances in which it is needed for insurance purposes or third parties. Further, Nancy McWilliams (1999) points towards one of the complexities of diagnosis with her observation that diagnosis becomes more difficult as therapy progresses and the therapist gets to know the patient better. It is much easier to provide an objective diagnosis of a patient in the first session rather than the tenth session.

"Careful about diagnostic labels. You are working with people who often do not fit nicely into a category."

To this end, it is also useful to consider that *therapy* and *assessment* are two different constructs and practices. Therapy typically involves rapport building, understanding, and collaboration. Inherent to this process is subjectivity. Conversely, assessment is typified by objectivity and a less-involved working relationship. The focus of assessment is a specific question, such as whether the patient meets diagnostic criteria for a condition. Engagement is typically shorter and the referral reason or presenting problem is clearly defined with strict parameters.

Diagnosis and its application represent an ever-changing field. It can be contentious, with differing views about the inclusion of particular diagnoses in the DSM (American Psychiatric Association, 2013) and other diagnostic manuals. This pertains to diagnostic criteria, public demand for diagnosis, public understanding of diagnosis and its consequences, and expectations and regulations from funders and insurance bodies. Therapists should be mindful of reactivity to public sentiment regarding diagnosis. This includes maintaining a mindful position of their own training, expertise, competence, and capacity in response to public demand.

Public sentiment and professional opinion about diagnosis and specific diagnoses will change over time. An astute therapist will be mindful of this, while adhering to their professional obligations and ensuring their practice remains within the scope of their training and expertise. To this end, diagnosis should always be a collaborative and consensual exercise. Informed consent for the patient is part of this – the therapist must ensure the patient is aware of the potential benefits, limitations, and consequences or diagnostic assessment and its outcomes.

The following points may be useful for therapists to consider regarding diagnosis:

- Therapists should never feel pressured to diagnose a patient, or to confirm a self-diagnosis that a patient has derived from other sources, such as online information or via social media.
- Therapists must be careful to adhere to practice that is within their scope of competence, including conducting assessments. Some assessments require specific and specialised training in order to administer psychometric measurements and interpret scores and results.
- Therapists should consider their qualifications and competence in making a diagnosis.
- Always consider differential diagnosis. That is, look beyond the initial referral reason to consider other explanations for the patient's presentation. Patients may present with a query regarding a specific diagnosis, such as ADHD, however, it is imperative that a thorough assessment be conducted that considers other explanations for the patient's presentation.
- Patients are experts on their own lives, but through training and experience therapists hold expertise on assessment and diagnosis. A collaborative approach is therefore best.
- Consider the intended purpose of diagnosis. If a diagnostic report is requested or produced, be mindful that this may precipitate the therapist being called upon to give further information in contexts such as a court of law, or through third party communications such as insurance agencies. Therapists need to ensure they are working within their own scope of competence and training when writing reports that may be used for psycho-legal purposes, or for cases in which the report writer may be required to provide evidence as an expert witness.
- Consider that diagnosis is a dynamic concept. The suitability of a diagnosis for individuals may change over time, as symptoms change in terms of worsening or resolving. Further, our understanding and application of diagnosis changes over time; for example, the DSM (American Psychiatric Association, 2013) undergoes significant revisions each few years.

When working with individuals seeking diagnosis, therapists must provide informed consent around diagnostic assessment, including its potential risks and benefits. This is similar to the informed consent necessary for therapy services (see Chapter 2), but should also include information pertaining to:

- Estimate of costs (including cost per session, cost of written report).
- Estimate of anticipated number of sessions required to conduct assessment.
- Intended purpose of the diagnosis (i.e., personal knowledge, funding, referral for treatment).
- Communication of assessment results/diagnosis to the patient (i.e., verbal feedback, written report, or both).
- The possible impact of the diagnosis on the therapeutic relationship and attainment of therapeutic goals.
- Limits of the assessment and diagnosis. Therapists may specifically state that a diagnostic report is not to be considered for medicolegal purposes, such as insurance claims or other legal processes.
- Last, therapists should consider their own personal and professional biases in diagnoses. Some therapists are well-known for endorsing specific diagnoses or diagnosing the majority of their patients with one disorder, such as borderline personality or ADHD. In these instances, it is pertinent for the therapist to consider their own experiences of countertransference and how this may be impacting their capacity for objectivity and fair assessment. When all you have is a hammer, everything tends to look like a nail.

Summary

- Competence refers to the therapist's capacity to effectively and efficiently complete the tasks required of their role.
- Competence is a dynamic process. It is influenced by many factors, not least of which is the interaction between the therapist and patient.
- Competence can be measured objectively against a set of criteria, including knowledge, skills, and ethical and professional behaviour and practice.
- Therapists must always be mindful of working within their scope of competence, training, and expertise.
- Imposter syndrome refers to feelings of self-doubt around one's capacity and feelings of academic or professional fraudulence. While not a recognised diagnostic term, this phenomenon is common to trainee and early-career therapists.

- Imposter syndrome impacts therapists' professional and personal sense of self. It is associated with compassion fatigue and can precipitate burnout. Therapists experiencing imposter syndrome are therefore encouraged to adopt an introspective position, rather than push away or deny these difficult thoughts.
- Pertinent issues related to competence include selecting an area of expertise and choosing a therapeutic modality. These decisions can be aided by engaging in mentoring, completing a variety of professional development activities and workshops, and engaging as a patient in different therapy types.
- Therapists are encouraged to be especially mindful of their own competence and its limits when working with novel presentations or new patient populations.
- Diagnosis presents another area in which the therapist must be mindful of working within their scope of competence.

Reference list

American Psychiatric Association. (2013). *Diagnostic and statistical manual of mental disorders* (5th ed.). American Psychiatric Association.

Barnett, J. E., Zimmerman, J., & Walfish, S. (2014). *The ethics of private practice: A practical guide for mental health clinicians.* Oxford University Press.

Beck, J. S., & Beck, A. T. (1995). *Cognitive therapy: Basics and beyond.* Guilford Press.

Clance, P. R., & Imes, S. A. (1978). The imposter phenomenon in high achieving women: Dynamics and therapeutic intervention. *Psychotherapy: Theory, Research & Practice, 15*(3), 241–247. https://doi.org/10.1037/h0086006

Clark, P., Holden, C., Russell, M., & Downs, H. (2022). The imposter phenomenon in mental health professionals: Relationships among compassion fatigue, burnout, and compassion satisfaction. *Contemporary Family Therapy, 44,* 185–197. https://doi.org/10.1007/s10591-021-09580-y

Cozolino, L. (2004). *The making of a therapist.* Norton.

DeCandia Vitoria, A. (2021). Experiential supervision: Healing imposter phenomenon from the inside out. *The Clinical Supervisor, 40*(2), 200–217. https://doi.org/10.1080/07325223.2020.1830215

Denny, B. (2023, November 9). Self-diagnosis is on the rise, but is TikTok really to blame? *The Age.*

Frankcom, K., Stevens, B., & Watts, P. (2016). *Fit to practice.* Australian Academic Press.

Hackney, H. L., & Cormier, S. (2012). *The professional counselor: A process guide to helping* (7th ed.). Pearson.

McWilliams, N. (1999). *Psychoanalytical case formulation*. Guilford Press.

Türkel, N. N., Başaran, A. S., Gazey, H., & Ertek, İ. E. (2025). The imposter phenomenon in psychiatrists: Relationships among compassion fatigue, burnout, and maladaptive perfectionism. *BMC Psychiatry, 25*(1), 30. https://doi.org/10.1186/s12888-025-06470-7

Yalom, I. D. (2009). *The gift of therapy: Reflections on being a therapist*. Harper Perennial.

Notes, reports, and record-keeping

7

The work of a therapist comes with a hefty amount of paperwork and administration. Notes, reports, and record-keeping are essential tasks. While this work occurs "behind the scenes" and typically out of the view of patients and colleagues, administrative tasks should never be considered an afterthought. These are fundamental components of being a therapist. Notes, reports, and record-keeping inform and facilitate the face-to-face aspects of therapy.

Some therapists bemoan administrative tasks. Many envision therapy work to be solely face-to-face contact with patients. In reality, upwards of 30% of a therapist's work time will be spent on non-patient facing tasks. For therapists, there is really no escaping administrative aspects of work; while some administration and paperwork can be outsourced, therapists remain responsible to ensure tasks are completed in a manner that is consistent with ethical and professional standards. Each step of working with patients must be contemporaneously documented and stored in an appropriate and secure manner. Therefore, therapists who feel they are not "administratively minded" are encouraged to adopt strategies and develop skills in this area. Like with any learned behaviour, confidence and competence around administrative tasks improves with attention, practice, and time.

Notes, reports, and patient records comprise the bulk of the therapist's administrative workload. Other tasks may include telephone calls, billing and invoicing, and scheduling. Therapists must be able to demonstrate competence and compliance in relation to administrative tasks, particularly related to the three main area of notes, reports, and patient records (Barnett et al., 2014).

DOI: 10.4324/9781003533030-7

Notes

All contact with patients must be recorded in the form of session notes. Notes need to be accurate, complete, and up to date. Adequate notes best support the interests of patients, while also protecting the therapist by demonstrating that the work with the patient was appropriate and completed to an expected standard.

Notes provide a primary record of treatment. While the purpose of notes varies dependent on the reader of said notes, there are generally three important stakeholders to consider: therapists, patients, and registration boards or regulatory bodies. For therapists, notes provide a memory jog or memorandum for session content, allowing continuity of care by enabling session planning, and informing case conceptualisation or formulation. For patients, notes provide a summary of their clinical information. For registration boards or regulatory bodies (in the case of patient complaints or other disciplinary matters), notes provide evidence of the therapist's thinking, planning, and adherence to responsibilities around delivery of treatment that is ethically sound and evidence-based.

"Take the time to develop good note-taking skills
and to have a loose plan for the next session."

Notes are subjective. There is no one set formula or standard format that must be adhered to. Therapists will find their own style over time; however, novice therapists invariably find templates and pro-forma documents helpful for guidance. These provide useful structure and a guide to the type and amount of information to be included.

The essential components of patient notes include:

- Date and time
- Place of treatment (i.e., consulting room, telehealth session)
- Session number
- Persons present
- Nature of session (i.e., initial, assessment, therapy, termination session)
- Mental Status Examination (MSE)
- Content of session
- Date of next session
- Brief plan for next session
- Name and signature of therapist, with date (and co-signature of supervisor, if applicable)

Notes are best organised in a way that reflects the structure of the session. Subheadings are useful to organise information and create a flow for ease of reading and comprehension. For example, subheadings for a session focused on social phobia may include *psychoeducation about social phobia*, *construction of exposure hierarchy*, or *setting homework*.

A Mental Status Examination (MSE) is essential to include in every session note. The purpose of an MSE is to provide a contemporaneous indication of the patient's current presentation and well-being. This can then be used by the therapist (or others providing treatment) to track changes over time, such as deterioration of mood, changes in thinking patterns, or inattention to hygiene and grooming. Similar to other components of notes or patient records, the MSE can be used to communicate information to other therapists or health professionals with whom the patient interacts.

The four main components of an MSE are:

1. Mood and affect:
   - "Patient presents with euthymic mood and reactive affect."
2. Presentation and grooming:
   - "Patient presented to session dressed in jeans and T-shirt. Attire was appropriate to weather. Patient was neatly groomed, with attention to hair and make-up."
3. Thought content and speech:
   - "Patient's speech was pressured. Tangential, difficult to contain at times. No evidence or disordered thought content."
4. Risk:
   - "Patient reports increased suicidal ideation. No plan or intent reported."
   - Risk should always be noted, even if the absence of a formal risk assessment or any indication of harm to self or others. For example, "no risk of harm to self or others."

The type of amount of information to include in notes is a common point of concern for trainee and early-career therapists. Novice therapists are often anxious about missing information and hence include superfluous or excessive information.

Common questions from trainee and early-career therapists include:

- "How much detail should be included?"
- "How extensive should my notes be?"
- "What wording or language should be used?"
- "What information should or can be excluded?"

"You might write too much from fear of not writing enough."

Therapists must be selective and parsimonious with information. This is a skill that develops over time, and one that improves with practice. There is no need for a verbatim transcript of the session. Notes are a summary of a session and should not be a script or a "he said, she said" record of each word or thought expressed.

When writing notes, therapists should reflect on the main themes or key points of the therapy sessions; this helps with notes being comprehensible and also encourages the therapist to think in terms of the patient formulation and informs treatment planning.

Notes should be written in an active rather than passive voice. Facts, rather than opinion, are reported. For example, "John reported his boss to be verbally aggressive", rather than "John's boss is verbally aggressive".

Notes are usually confidential; however, there is always a possibility that these may be read by patients, or that they may be requested for insurance or legal reasons. Notes should be written with this in mind – avoid unnecessary information and exclude names and unessential details of other people who may be discussed in therapy sessions. Be brief and direct, with a clear focus on the presenting problem and reason for referral. Write notes in plain language, in a manner that would allow patients and other parties to gauge a general understanding of the content.

"Use an active voice. Be clear about what the patient themselves has said, what is your opinion, and what is your observation."

Insufficient, inaccurate, or incomplete notes is a common area of difficulty for therapists facing disciplinary action by registration boards or licensing bodies (Frankcom et al., 2016). Completing notes in a timely and accurate manner is important to promote good practice; this acts as a protective mechanism for both therapists and patients in the instance of complaints or disciplinary action. Keep all notes in such a manner that they will be held up to scrutiny if challenged. Memory and recall are unreliable, but contemporaneous notes provide a consistent and dependable record of events.

Effective and efficient note-keeping

Effective and efficient note-keeping is a common challenge for trainee and early-career therapists. Novice therapists are prone to excessively long or overly detailed notes. They often spend an excessive amount of time on notes, leading to a glut of unfinished notes. This can be anxiety-provoking and distressing for therapists, with many feeling they have little choice but to spend copious out-of-work hours catching up on session notes.

The personality characteristics common to therapists – including perfectionism, rigidity of thinking, and attention to detail – seem to promote these difficulties with note-keeping (Cozolino, 2004). Therapists are encouraged to think about their own personal qualities and how these impact the efficiency and effectiveness of note-keeping. This can be due to characteristics of the therapist (such as perfectionism) or a tendency on the therapist's behalf to over-complicate the task of note-keeping. From a practical perspective, some therapists struggle with keeping up to date with notes due to not calculating this task as an essential part of their workload or time allocation. At a process level, difficulties with note-keeping can reflect a problem within the therapy itself, including a lack of organisation or structure within the therapy session, or a lack of clarity around the formulation or treatment plan. In addition to personal reflection, supervision can be a useful space to discuss note-keeping. Difficulties with efficient and effective note-keeping can be reflective of other concerns.

Most trainee and early-career therapists take "scratch notes" while in session with patients. This information is then used to inform the writing up of a final session note that is stored on the patient's file. Scratch notes are a useful way to gather information, particularly for novice therapists who worry about forgetting important points or essential information. When taking notes in session, it is imperative to balance gathering information with rapport building and need to connect with patients; be mindful of maintaining eye contact and observing nonverbal aspects of patients' behaviour, such as mood and affect.

---

*"You will find your style in note-taking and
it will all come together."*

Therapists tend to take fewer notes as they gain experience and develop confidence around their capacity to remember information. Over time, therapists develop the skill of discerning superfluous information and unnecessary details. An experienced therapist will glean information that is useful to inform formulation and understanding of the patient and their presenting problem. Understandably, this skill takes time to develop. Practice and exposure to a variety of sessions and patients will facilitate the development of these skills. Further, adopting specific strategies can be helpful in establishing good practices around this essential area of work.

"You need peace of mind that your practices around notes are sufficiently watertight, so you can devote your energy to working and not worrying about such an essential part of the frame."

Strategies to promote efficient and effective note-keeping include:

1. Proformas and templates.
   Proformas and templates provide useful prompts for content, together with the amount of information to include in each section. These are readily available and often provided by training programmes. There are many different formats, based on session type (i.e., intake, assessment, therapy), and patient population (i.e., child, adult, couples, family). Therapists can also construct their own templates and pro-formas.

"I have templates for all my notes. I spend 5–10 mins max on session notes."

---

2. Be parsimonious with information.
   Write less. This is a simple and effective strategy, but for many trainee and early-career therapists, it is easier said than done. Good notes are concise, clear, and comprehensive. Long-winded notes are often a reflection of lack of discernment around clinical information.

   Parsimonious writing is a skill that can be practised. Similar to cutting words from an essay or other piece of writing, therapists can practise this skill by editing their own notes. Set a word limit or page limit, then work towards achieving that.

   For example:

   John is a 45-year-old man. He is married to Sue, and they have two children. Sam is 14 years old and in year 9 at high school. Katie is 16 years old and in year 11 at high school. They have a dog, Millie.

John works as a cleaner for the council. He likes his job. A few weeks ago, John slipped over on a piece of plastic at work. He fell over and hurt his knee.

John has been feeling horrible lately. He says he has a racing heart and sweaty palms. John has been sleeping for only 4 hours each night and is tired during the day at work.

Can be summarised to:

John is a 45-year-old man, married to Sue, with two teenage children (Sam and Katie). John recently experienced a workplace incident in his role as a cleaner at the municipal council, in which he fell and sustained a knee injury. Since this time, he has experienced physiological symptoms of anxiety, in addition to irritability and insomnia.

3. Set a timer.

   Use a timer to allocate an amount of time to complete notes. The amount of time can be modified, as experience and skills around notewriting become more refined.

   This experiment can be tailored to the individual therapist. For novice therapists, a time limit of 20 minutes to complete a session note may be reasonable. When time is up, evaluate the type and amount of content completed. Reflect on any unnecessary or superfluous information and consider how the time could be used in a different way. This strategy encourages the therapist to prioritise including essential information and will alert them to areas in which there are challenges in writing briefly and succinctly.

4. Complete notes as soon as possible.

   Notes are best completed as soon as possible after each therapy session. Many experienced therapists run 50-minute sessions and complete their session notes in the remaining 10 minutes of the hour.

   Information is best recalled in the immediate time following a session. Always complete notes on the day of the session; this is a professional and ethical responsibility, but it also ensures that notes accurately reflect the content of the session.

   Allocating time within one's workday to complete notes is essential. Notes are not an afterthought but are instead an essential part of the patient session. The therapeutic work with a patient is not complete until all tasks related to the session are finalised. This includes notes.

5. Set a goal or reward.

   Human behaviour is best encouraged by positive reinforcement. In the absence of motivation to complete notes, structure is helpful. Related to notes, this could equate to not leaving the clinic or workplace until all notes are finished, or to delaying sending an invoice for the session until all notes are completed. Of course, the patient is not concerned with notes and will not be privy to the time frame around this task. But this provides an internal check and balance, for completing notes has a benefit to patients in terms of optimal clinical practice and good therapeutic care.

6. Write notes with the assumption that patients will read them.

Notes are generally confidential; however, there is always a chance that notes will be accessed by a patient or third party, such as for legal or insurance purposes. Always assume that patients will read the notes of their session, and write out the information accordingly. This will encourage plain language and avoidance of technical or long-winded terminology.

"Remember that notes could be read by anyone. How would you feel if your patient read in five years' time what you are writing about them today?"

Reports

For therapists, reports are a broad term encompassing several types of documents. Specifically, these include assessment reports and treatment reports (Pelling & Burton, 2018).

Reports are used to inform decision-making around diagnosis, intervention, and treatment. Reports are also used to inform a variety of other important decisions, such as those in educational, legal, and social contexts. Therapists are held in high regard in these settings; reports and the recommendations contained within them can have significant implications. It is therefore incumbent upon therapists to understand the nature of report writing. Therapists must ensure their report writing is consistent with their expertise and knowledge, and within the scope of their competence.

Assessment reports are completed for a specific purpose, such as providing diagnostic clarity, to gain understanding of a presenting problem, or to answer a specific referral question.

Assessment reports typically comprise four main sections (Pelling & Burton, 2018):

1. Background information:
   a. Reason for referral
   b. Presenting problem
   c. Relevant personal and psychological history

2. Assessment information:
   a. Preliminary consideration of symptoms
   b. Risk assessment
   c. Observations
   d. Assessment tools, psychometric measures
   e. Findings
3. Diagnosis:
   a. Formulation
   b. Rationale for diagnosis
   c. Differential diagnosis
   d. Diagnosis
4. Recommendations:
   a. Intervention
   b. Onward referral

Treatment reports, also known as intervention reports, follow a similar structure. The purpose of a treatment report differs from an assessment report in that it is a summary of the therapeutic work or intervention that has been conducted with a patient.

Key sections of treatment reports include (Pelling & Burton, 2018):

1. Background information:
   a. Reason for referral
   b. Presenting problem
   c. Relevant personal and psychological history
2. Assessment information:
   a. Preliminary consideration of symptoms
   b. Risk assessment
   c. Observations
   d. Assessment tools, psychometric measures
   e. Findings
3. Diagnosis:
   a. Formulation
   b. Rationale for diagnosis
   c. Differential diagnosis
   d. Diagnosis
4. Intervention:
   a. Plan
   b. Rationale for recommended intervention
   c. Implementation
   d. Evaluation

Both assessment reports and intervention reports must be dated and must carry the therapists' name, credentials, and signature. Reports by trainees and interns are typically co-signed by supervisors or other senior therapists.

Responding to requests for reports

Therapists often receive unsolicited requests for reports. Requests may come directly from patients (or their parents or caregivers), or from third parties such as a lawyers or insurance companies. Some reports may be mandatory to complete, such as a treatment plan or progress report from an insurer, but many requests are just that – requests. Therapists need to be discerning regarding this; third parties may present a request for a report in a manner that implies it is compulsory or urgent. Take the time to properly read the nature of the request, and to ensure it is within the scope of competence and is consistent with the nature of work being undertaken with the patient to whom the report applies.

The provision of a report should always be considered in the context of the best interests of the patient. Reports can have a significant impact on patients' well-being and prognosis, as reports are often considered in decision-making regarding aspects of care such as funding, eligibility for treatment, and special consideration for study and examinations.

Report writing is an essential task for therapists, and as such all therapists must demonstrate competence in the writing and comprehension of reports. However, some therapists are better placed to provide certain reports; this is based on factors such as experience, skill, and expertise. To this end, therapists should never feel pressured to provide a report that they judge to be outside of their scope of competence or knowledge. Further, therapists should never feel pressured to provide information or present a specific opinion or perspective. As always, seek supervision if further clarification is needed.

Therapists must reach a reasonable judgement regarding their competence and capacity to provide a requested report. In addition to their own professional attributes (knowledge, qualifications, skill), consideration for therapists includes:

- Identifying the subject/person of interest and evaluating your professional obligation to them
- Ascertaining the intended audience for a report (i.e., therapist, judiciary, funding body, school or University)

- Ascertaining the referral reason or question (i.e., prognosis, diagnosis, capacity for work, parenting capacity, funding for educational aide, legal proceedings, sentencing considerations, funding for school, special consideration for studies or exams)

Patient records

Record-keeping is essential to ensure competent, ethical, and effective treatment. Good business practice also relies on stringent and accurate record-keeping. Poor record-keeping leaves therapists vulnerable to patient complaints and difficulties with registration boards and licensing bodies (Barnett et al., 2014; Frankcom et al., 2016).

Also known as a patient file, a patient record is a collection of all documents relevant to a patient and the therapeutic care provided to them. The format of a patient record, together with the type and amount of information required, is usually specified by workplaces and organisations. The type and amount of information is also specific to individual workplaces; however, this must be consistent with legislation and regulatory requirements. Therapists working in private settings must also comply with legislation and regulatory requirements in the organisation and management of patient records. Each therapist will arrive at their own preference for patient files. This will vary dependent on patient population, workplace, and theoretical orientation.

A patient record is typically categorised into key sections. Whether the record is paper-based or an electronic file, it is arranged in a way that ensures information is clear and accessible. Information within each section is typically stored in chronological order.

Key sections and minimum requirements for patient records are outlined in Table 7.1. Some information is likely to be relevant to more than one section. Consistency is key here, with the main priority being that all information is organised and stored in a secure and accessible format. In deciding whether information should be stored in the "correspondence" or "notes" section, it is useful to remember that *correspondence* refers to things that are sent and received in a static manner (such as letters), while *notes* typically include dynamic interactions (such as telephone calls or patient sessions).

Beyond the essential information and minimum requirements previously noted, it may be appropriate to include further specific documents, such as a genogram. This is a visual representation of the family system in which the patient operates. It is a visual diagram used to represent

Table 7.1 Patient records sections and minimum requirements.

Signed informed consent document(s)	Informed consent must be obtained prior to undertaking any therapeutic work with a patient. This includes information related to confidentiality, storage and release of information, and policies related to fees and other administrative matters. Informed consent is further detailed in Chapter 2.
Correspondence	Therapists typically obtain various correspondence in the course of working with a patient. This may include referral letters, legal requests, and communication from other therapists or health professionals. Reports (including those written by the therapist and those composed by others) would also be stored in this section. All correspondence – including that received via email or other electronic means – must be stored in the patient file.
Notes	Contemporaneous notes must be made for each session with a patient. Other patient-related events should also be documented, with notes stored in the patient file. These may include minutes of case conference meetings, communication with a patient's parents or caregivers, or details of telephone conversations.
Psychometric measures and test results	Documents related to any testing conducted with a patient must be collated and stored in the patient record. This includes raw data, such as scoring sheets and response booklets.

and understand systemic relationships, usually among family members. This therapist's version of a "family tree" also provides detail on the interactions between members, such as alliances and estrangements. Genograms adopt conventions and symbols to indicate life events such as divorce and deaths, making them a useful short-hand for therapists to refer to as a reminder of the patient's life and history (Hackney & Cormier, 2012).

Other sections may be included within the patient file, including those to store information and documents such as scratch notes (notes taken during a session), records of supervision related to the patient, formulation notes, and information related to billing and invoicing.

Notes and record-keeping practices will vary by setting.
Keep this in mind when developing your own style.

Storage and destruction of patient records

Strict rules and regulations apply to the storage and disposal of all information and documents pertaining to therapy patients, including patient records. Respect for patient confidentiality is paramount in the storage of records, just as it is at every stage of therapy. All patient records must be stored in a secure manner. As part of the informed consent process, patients are made aware of the way in which their information is stored, including requirements about the length of time that records may be maintained (Australian Psychological Society, 2020).

Paper records must be stored in locked filing cabinets, with keys stored away from cabinets. Filing cabinets should ideally be located in a separate lockable room accessible only to those with authority to retrieve and access patient records (Barnett et al., 2014). A registry facility can be used to indicate records that are removed either temporarily (such as for a patient session) or permanently (such as for purposes or archiving or disposal). Filing cabinets should be arranged to promote ease of access to information, including sections for current patients and archived records. Noting the date of the last contact on archived records can be useful to indicate the date after which the record may be destroyed.

Paper records should never be left unattended, nor taken off-site. These leave patient information open to the risk of confidentiality breaches. To this end, session notes should be completed contemporaneously – that is, all notes and work related to a patient session should be completed at the workplace and on the day of the session, rather than taken home or to another place to be completed.

Never alter or tamper with a note after the date on which it was initially written; a brief explanatory addendum section can be added should information need to be amended or clarified. All notes must feature signature and date, or an electronic time-stamp.

In the digital age, many therapists utilise electronic devices or cloud-based services for notes and patient records. Regardless of whether information is stored in paper or electronic format, the therapist remains responsible for safeguarding patients' information and protecting patient confidentiality. For electronic records, therapists are responsible for ensuring that storage of information complies with current national standards for health data and patient information (Australian Psychological Society, 2020). Typically, it is not necessary to retain paper copies of documents that have been scanned and stored in electronic format. Any scans must be legible and true copies of original documents.

Further considerations related to electronic records include:

- Electronic systems or software used to store records must be compliant with legislation.
- Information is stored and categorised in relation to levels of accessibility (i.e., clinical records may be accessed only by authorised users such as therapists, while administrative staff can access general patient information and billing information).
- Information is encrypted in accordance with legislative requirements.
- Information is password protected. Passwords are regularly updated.

Time frames for storage of patient records vary between jurisdictions and professions. This is typically stated in legislation related to health records, and more clearly explicated by professional organisations and regulatory bodies. For example, in Australia, patient records must be retained for seven years from the point of last clinical contact or until the patient is 25 years old. Further, there is specific legislation related to the storage of records for First Nations and Indigenous patients, together with those participating in therapy as part of government redress or compensation schemes, such as in relation to forced adoption or institutional abuse (Australian Institute of Health and Welfare, 2010). It is the responsibility of each therapist to maintain current knowledge of record-keeping requirements, particularly around specific patient populations for whom records may need to be kept for an extended period of time. Membership of a professional organisation or association can be useful in understanding and applying legislation, as information relevant to changes to patient records and record-keeping are often disseminated in the form of newsletters, bulletin board posts, or via electronic communication.

Individual organisations and workplaces may impose additional requirements on storage of patient records. As always, in the case of conflicting information between legislation requirements and workplace expectations, therapists are obliged to comply with legislation. In this case, therapists should seek supervision and discuss any concerns with their workplace.

Therapists must also pre-emptively consider record storage in case of their incapacitation or death. This is particularly pertinent for therapists working in a private practice or clinic setting, where the therapist may manage some or all aspects of record-keeping. To this end, therapists should develop a professional will, in which instructions are stipulated for ongoing care of patients and management of other administrative considerations, including patient records (American Psychological Association, 2014; Australian Psychological Society, 2021). A colleague is nominated to manage communication with patients, including requests for information and requests for access to notes and records. Further information related to professional wills and therapists' responsibility to ensure continuity of patient care in the event of incapacitation or death is contained in Chapter 11.

**

The appropriate disposal of patient information is equally as important as appropriate storage. Disposing of patient information presents a risky time for breaches of patient confidentiality; old records may be accessed and moved for the first time in many years, perhaps leading the therapist to leave a filing cabinet unlocked or place files in a car or other place before fulfilling an intention to dispose of the documents.

All information – both paper and electronic – must be disposed of in a safe and permanent manner. Before doing so, it is useful to retain a list of names and dates for future reference; this can be helpful if information is requested by a patient or third party after the patient records have been destroyed (Corey et al., 2024). Even the most well-meaning and conscientious therapist cannot rely on memory to recall names and dates of all patients. A concise record therefore provides clear information for individual patients and third parties (such as lawyers or insurance companies). This will put the therapist's mind at ease regarding the existence and location of patient records.

Paper copies must be disposed in a way that is permanent and does not allow for any access to information. It is never sufficient to place paper records in a household or commercial garbage receptacle. All records must be *completely* destroyed, with no information decipherable. Shredding provides a reliable disposal process. Ripping pages by hand or cutting using scissors is not acceptable. Workplaces (such as hospitals and clinics) have shredding machines or secure repositories for the disposal of confidential or sensitive documents. Private waste disposal companies and office-supply stores also offer commercial shredding services; these can be useful for larger quantities of paper records or for those therapists who do not have access to a shredder.

Summary

- All therapists must demonstrate competence in administrative tasks, including notes, reports, and record-keeping.
- Each session and patient interaction must be contemporaneously documented. These session notes are a primary record of treatment, containing essential information pertaining to the patient, course of treatment, and treatment outcomes.
- Efficient, accurate, and parsimonious notes is a common challenge for trainee and early-career therapists. Strategies for effective note-keeping include setting time limits, writing notes as soon as possible following a session, practising summarising information, and setting goals and rewards.
- Report writing is a key skill for all therapists, including assessment reports and treatment reports. As in all aspects of practice, therapists must be mindful of working within their scope of competence in relation to providing reports regarding particular patient populations, diagnoses, and specific areas of practice.
- Records must be maintained for all patients. A patient record is a collection of all documents relevant to a patient and the therapeutic care in which they have engaged.
- Confidentiality is paramount to all aspects of record-keeping. Patient records must be stored in a secure manner, whether paper-based or electronic.
- Patient records must be stored for a set period of time, as indicated by legislation and privacy laws. Permanent destruction of records (via shredding of paper documents or permanent deletion of electronic files) can occur only after this designated period of time.

Reference list

American Psychological Association. (2014). *Your professional will: Why and how to create.* https://www.apaservices.org/practice/good-practice/professional-will-instructions.pdf

Australian Institute of Health and Welfare. (2010). *National best practice guidelines for collecting Indigenous status in health data sets.* AIHW.

Australian Psychological Society. (2020). *Record keeping in organisations.* https://psychology.org.au/getmedia/ed4030cc-d8f3-478f-b94a-975a5b59893c/20aps-position-statement-record-keeping-p1.pdf

Australian Psychological Society. (2021). Understanding practice contingency plans. *InPsych, 43(3)*.

Barnett, J. E., Zimmerman, J., & Walfish, S. (2014). *The ethics of private practice: A practical guide for mental health clinicians*. Oxford University Press.

Corey, G., Corey, M. S., & Corey, C. (2024). *Issues & ethics in the helping professions* (11th ed.). Cengage.

Cozolino, L. (2004). *The making of a therapist*. Norton.

Frankcom, K., Stevens, B., & Watts, P. (2016). *Fit to practice*. Australian Academic Press.

Hackney, H. L., & Cormier, S. (2012). *The professional counselor: A process guide to helping* (7th ed.). Pearson.

Pelling, N., & Burton, L. J. (Eds.). (2018). *The elements of psychological case report writing in Australia*. Routledge.

Transference and countertransference   **8**

Trainee and early-career therapists tend to be rattled by the psychological phenomena of transference and countertransference. In my own training and in that described by my colleagues, the concepts of transference and countertransference were considered "too advanced" or complex for novice therapists to understand or apply. I have wondered whether this was about shielding novice therapists from difficult content, or moreover a product of senior therapists wanting to elevate themselves by reserving knowledge. Regardless, the processes of transference and countertransference occur independently of a therapist's (or patient's) understanding of them, just as the temperature is felt by someone who has no knowledge or understanding of the scales of temperature measured by Celsius or Fahrenheit.

Novice therapists can and should have an understanding of transference and countertransference. These concepts can seem complicated, but they are not beyond the understanding of therapists, who learn and apply similarly complex knowledge and skills throughout their training and work. An understanding of these concepts will allow further learning of more complex notions associated with these psychological phenomena.

Many a supervisee has confided concerns related to *feeling* something towards their patient. Others have reported surprise at being told by patients that the therapist has been in their thoughts outside of sessions, perhaps through daydreams or dreams. Understandably, this can represent an unusual or unsettling experience for therapists who are very much focused on being in the room with patients, rather than thinking about the deeper sequalae of the therapeutic relationship. Therapists sometimes fret about how to respond to these experiences, often pondering whether thinking or

DOI: 10.4324/9781003533030-8

feeling something about a patient (and vice versa) represents a breach of the therapeutic violation.

> *"Don't be put off by all the technical language that*
> *can make psychodynamic therapy spookier than it is."*

Rest assured, it is *completely normal* to feel some kind of emotional reaction towards patients. Therapists are human beings sitting in front of another human being (Jung, 1946). From that perspective, it would be odd if therapists *did not* have some kind of emotional response to patients.

Rather than be a matter of concern, this realisation from supervisees is to be celebrated. It often demonstrates an advance in thinking and clinical skill; wondering about transference (even if the phenomena have not yet been labelled or understood) usually indicates understanding of and command over the foundational skills of therapy. This shows that the therapist has integrated essential skills. They are adopting an advanced perspective and deeper thinking; space has opened up in which the therapist can consider not only the *content* of therapy (the words and stories of patients), but also the *process*. It is within the *process* of therapy – that is, how the therapist and patient relate to each other and the feelings each evoke in the other – that therapeutic change is essentially enacted (Yalom, 1989).

Essentially, therapists and their patients each have their own history, unresolved conflicts, assumptions about the world, thoughts, and feelings; the interaction of these – or the way they *transfer* between therapist and patient – impacts the way therapy progresses and shapes the attainment of therapeutic goals.

> *"Transference means the relationship templates our brains*
> *carry around, formed elsewhere and earlier, which they use*
> *to guess what the person in front of you will do next. It*
> *happens all the time, so that we get a moment-by-moment,*
> *feeling-driven guide of how to act."*

The topic of transference sparks much conjecture and lively debate in academic circles. Entire books, journal series, and conferences are dedicated to it. Some therapists and theorists devote their lives to studying and writing about it. There is some academic acquiescence around its core definition and components; however, this deeply intriguing phenomenon continues to attract divergent understandings from proponents of different therapeutic modalities and schools.

Keeping these complexities in mind, it is entirely sufficient for trainee and early-career therapists to gain an understanding of the basic premise of transference and countertransference and a general overview of the implications of these for therapeutic practice. Further knowledge can be gained in later career stages.

Understanding transference and countertransference

First, a brief history of the term. Its origins have been attributed to Sigmund Freud, who first used the term to communicate his view that important feelings about adults in early childhood are "transferred" or cast onto others (Yalom, 2009).

Transference and related terms were traditionally the domains of psychoanalytical psychotherapy and psychodynamic psychotherapy. These psychological phenomena are deemed central to both these modalities, and each developed detailed and nuanced views on transference and its implications. As such, transference and countertransference are core to the education and training around these therapeutic modalities.

"It's never about the thing."

More recently, the understanding and use of transference and countertransference have been generalised and applied to other therapeutic modalities. The terms are now more commonly understood and discussed in the education and training of all therapists. An awareness of the concept and its impact is useful for all therapists regardless of therapeutic modality. The main types of transference are summarised in Table 8.1.

Transference

Transference occurs when a patient projects onto their therapist the feelings, experiences, or attitudes held towards significant people in their life (Gabbard, 2005). This represents a misattribution; the patient is not consciously aware that they are bringing a previous experience to the current therapeutic relationship.

Table 8.1 Main types of transference.

Transference	Patients project onto their therapist the past feelings, experiences, or attitudes they hold towards significant people in their lives.
Countertransference	Therapists project onto their patients the past feelings, experiences, or attitudes they hold towards significant people in their lives.
Co-transference	Encompasses both transference and countertransference.
Erotic transference	Patients' feelings of romantic or sexual attraction developed towards the therapist.

Essentially, transference is a term used to describe the past repeating itself in the present. Instead of overtly remembering or acknowledging the past, the patient unconsciously re-enacts past events and relational patterns (usually formed in childhood and early family experiences). From a neuroscience perspective, transference can be explained by the activation of neurons that trigger a memory (Corey et al., 2024; Gabbard, 2005).

"It of course gets tricky when we mistake our transference for actual knowledge of the person in front of us. That's why looking back on an interaction afterwards can be useful – what was them and what was me?"

Table 8.2 Common examples of transference.

Type	Definition	Example
Paternal	Patient views the therapist as a father figure and attributes characteristics of their own father to the therapist.	The patient's father was authoritative and protective; these characteristics are also assumed to be held by the therapist.
Maternal	Patient views the therapist as a mother figure and attributes characteristics of their own mother to the therapist.	The patient's mother was stern and quick to anger; the patient "walks on eggshells" around the therapist, assuming they may evoke an angry response.

The process of transference can begin prior to the first meeting between therapist and patient. It may be shaped by general ideas of therapists in the media or in popular culture, knowledge of the individual therapist (from friends, referring doctor), and previous experiences of therapists (Gabbard, 2005).

Common examples of transference are summarised in Table 8.2. Transference may be categorised as positive or negative, with the broad categorisation based on the type of feeling projected onto the therapist.

Countertransference

Some patients remind therapists of experiences or relationships in their own lives. These relationships may be problematic or representative of difficult experiences. This can bring unresolved conflict – of which all therapists have – to the fore in the therapist's work with clients, through a concept called countertransference. Similar to transference, in which the patient projects onto the therapist, countertransference occurs when the therapist projects onto patients past feelings, experiences, or attitudes they hold towards significant people in their lives (Cozolino, 2004).

Examples of this may include a therapist assuming older male patients to be angry or aggressive, based on their own paternal experiences, or a therapist whose own concerns about fertility lead them to give extra attention towards a pregnant patient.

*"The most important thing you can take
into the room is self-awareness."*

Trainee and early-career therapists often bristle at the idea of countertransference, assuming it to be negative. However, when recognised and managed, countertransference can be productive and constructive. The therapist's thoughts and feelings are a source of valuable information about the patient's relationships and internal world (Barnett et al., 2014).

Working with countertransference is at the core of several relational psychotherapy modalities, including psychodynamic psychotherapy and relational psychoanalysis. In these modalities, close attention is paid to the relationship and interactions between therapists and patients. In this sense, therapists' feelings towards patients can be used to inform the formulation about patients, particularly around interpersonal dynamics and their behaviour and experiences within interpersonal relationships. A therapist's response to a patient is a valuable source of information; their feelings towards a patient (i.e., annoyance, irritability, sympathy, pity, disconnection) can give an indication of how other people in the patient's life may feel and respond towards them (Yalom, 2009). Here, the notion of the therapy session being a microcosm of the patient's world is illuminated and harnessed. The experience of dysfunctional themes and patterns being identified and modified in therapy can then be generalised by the patient to their lives and other relationships, with the goal of impacting change in the patient's life.

However, countertransference can be destructive when not accurately recognised or appropriately managed. This occurs when therapists' issues become entangled with patients' concerns, thus obstructing or destroying their objectivity (DeYoung, 2022). For this reason, it is vital to build skills around identifying and managing countertransference.

"Things that don't make sense can sometimes be made sense of through the lens of transference."

Co-transference

The term "co-transference" was coined by psychoanalyst and psychoanalytic theorist Donna Orange (1995). The single term of co-transference encompasses both transference and countertransference and refers to the patient's general reactions to the therapist and the therapist's reactions in response. It emphasises the *interaction* of all that is in the minds of therapists and patients. This term strongly reflects a contemporary relational psychotherapy approach, in which the intersubjectivity between therapists and patients is held paramount to treatment and its outcomes (Pocock, 2006).

Erotic transference

Erotic transference, also referred to as sexualised transference, occurs when a patient feels overwhelmed with desire for a therapist. The patient may wish to pursue a romantic relationship or engage in sexual activity with their therapist. These feelings may be indicated by the patient in an overt manner or subtle ways. This is an unconscious process; the patient experiences the feelings of attraction as genuine (McWilliams, 1999).

Erotic transference is more complex than a patient simply finding their therapist physically attractive or sexually desirable. It can be understood in the same way as the general concept of transference – that is, the patient's relational patterns or past experiences are being brought into the current therapeutic relationship.

Similarly, sometimes therapists will experience erotic countertransference. Again, this is beyond finding a patient attractive. An important distinction exists between finding a patient attractive, being attracted to a patient, and experiencing limerence or a preoccupation with a patient. Transient feelings of sexual attraction are normal, but preoccupation with clients is problematic (Barnett et al., 2014).

The tendency to treat erotic transference as taboo (just as many issues related to sex and intimacy remain taboo within society) contributes to and compounds challenges faced by patients and therapists experiencing erotic transference. The resulting embarrassment or fear of reprisal can deter therapists from openly discussing these issues with colleagues or during supervision. More open acknowledgement of this experience and an understanding between sexual attraction and erotic transference is needed to counter this stigma.

Feelings arising from erotic transference must never be acted upon. A therapist must never engage in any sexual activity with a patient. Erotic countertransference should be viewed as an indication of the therapist's unmet needs for intimacy. It may signal emptiness or dissatisfaction within their own relationships, and as such the therapist should reflect on the happenings in their own life and relationships that may be contributing to or creating the erotic countertransference (Cozolino, 2004). Supervision and personal therapy are useful to explore countertransference experiences, including erotic countertransference.

Working with patients who get under your skin

Therapists find some patients more difficult to work with than others. Sometimes the cause of this is obvious; just like meeting an individual in a social setting, we quickly gather an idea of someone's likeability and our feelings towards the person. This may be informed by factors such as their interpersonal style, values and principles, and aspects of behaviour. Other times, the therapist may struggle to identify the impetus for the difficulty in the therapeutic relationship. In these instances, the therapist needs to delve a little deeper to understand their reaction to the patient, and to consider why a particular patient or presentation is getting under their skin.

No therapist is obliged to work with every single presentation or with all patients who have been referred to them. However, terminating a therapeutic relationship on the basis of personal dislike for a patient may not always be feasible. Discharging or refusing to work with a patient may not be consistent with an ethical approach or may fail to fulfil the therapist's duty of care. In some situations, the therapist must find a way forward in working with patients who they find difficult to work with.

Recognising one's own experience of and reaction to countertransference is integral to establishing and maintaining professional boundaries. At particularly stressful times of life, it may be prudent to decline to work with a particular patient population or presentation. This may be a recognition of a therapist's own unresolved conflict (which may be the focus of personal therapy) or a more acute response to current life circumstances.

Therapists are human, too. At particular times in their own lives, working with a patient experiencing similar life crises is likely to be difficult for the therapist. Examples of this include marriage breakdown or relationship difficulties, family violence, bereavement, and pregnancy loss or infertility. All therapists have scars and wounds; an effective therapist recognises this and works from the scar, not the wound.

Concepts related to transference are extremely important in psychotherapy. However, therapists must be wary of transference being used to explain everything (Gabbard, 2005). Be careful of incorrectly attributing all therapeutic processes and outcomes to transference and countertransference. A patient response may be entirely appropriate and represent an accurate and timely reflection of the current situation. For instance, a therapist who is running late may wish to explain a patient's annoyance at their tardiness by attributing this to being let down by caregivers early in life; while this exacerbates the patient's response, the therapist should also consider that annoyance at being left waiting is a normal and commensurate response.

Managing transference and countertransference

The first step in managing transference and countertransference is recognition. To do this, therapists need an understanding of themselves and their template of the world. This includes their own relational history, coping strategies, history of trauma or other significant life events, beliefs and assumptions, and biases against individuals or groups of people.

Transference and countertransference can feel like nebulous concepts. They can be difficult to understand, especially for trainee and early-career therapists who are also mastering a wide range of other skills. Therapists' skills around this improves with time, practice, and targeted supervision. The training and early-career stage is an opportune time for therapists to begin thinking about transference and countertransference, and to start discussions around these concepts in supervision. Imperative to this is curiosity about the self, and a willingness to learn about the self and others.

Self-awareness and understanding is imperative to recognising counter-transference (Hackney & Cormier, 2012). A starting point is to write a written reflection after each session. To begin, it may be useful to select one patient to focus on; learning about these concepts is an intense and sometimes fatiguing experience. Go slowly and allow yourself to be guided by supervisory support. Reviewing video and/or audio recordings can be useful to glean information.

Start with the question, "Where am I in this therapeutic relationship?" Some further questions may include the following:

- Am I feeling overprotective of this patient?
- Am I feeling more invested in this patient's progress, in comparison to my work with other patients?
- Am I being dismissive of the patient's concerns?
- Am I treating them in a benign or overly gentle manner?
- Am I setting different boundaries for this patient, or making different allowances for them? This may be loaning a personal book, offering an appointment outside of usual consulting hours, or charging a reduced fee.
- How do I feel *before* seeing this patient? This may include negative feelings (dread, fear, anxiety, worry) or positive feelings (excitement, anticipation).
- How do I feel when in the room *with* this patient? This may include feeling endangered, enlivened, emboldened, shy, recalcitrant, bored, tedious, or ill-equipped. Notice if this changes over the duration of the session, or between sessions.
- How does time pass during sessions with this patient? Does the time drag, or seem to go quickly? Do I lose track of time with this patient? Do I run late, or find my usual time management skills are difficult to apply?
- How do I feel *after* a session with this patient?
- Is this patient coming up in my thoughts and daydreams?
- Are any of these feelings familiar from my own history or relationships with other people?

Further, therapists need to be mindful of their own cultural assumptions. Ideas around parenting, relationships, education, and lifestyle behaviours (such as use of drugs and alcohol) are all heavily informed by personal history, values, beliefs, and assumptions (Cozolino, 2004). An oft-cited example of countertransference is Yalom's prescient observations of his own reaction to an overweight client; Yalom identified that his negative feelings towards the client and her larger size were due to his own assumptions about obesity being related to laziness, unproductivity, and ill health (Berman, 2019).

The "here and now" approach is one way for therapists to manage and use countertransference experiences (Yalom, 2009). Noticing countertransference in the moment is an ability that develops over time, just like other therapeutic skills. The therapist then uses the information garnered about the patient through countertransference to shape their interactions with the patient.

Burnout

Burnout is a slow and insidious process. Its progress can often go unnoticed and unchecked, until the therapist finds themselves in a state of complete exhaustion or a consequence of the burnout, such as an ethical transgression, is observed by others. A therapist experiencing burnout represents a position of professional compromise, as it typically impacts the therapist's ability to work in an ethical or competent manner.

Therapists experiencing burnout report that their work begins to feel laborious, stressful, or even painful. Physical ailments, such as headaches or intestinal problems, may be an indication of tension (Cozolino, 2004).

Inadequate or insufficient attention to issues of transference and countertransference can be a precursor to burnout. Therapists become consumed by patients and their needs, losing sight of their own well-being. Combined with the usual therapist characteristics of conscientiousness and, for some, perfectionism, issues related to transference and countertransference can be an unrecognised but significant contributing factor to burnout.

Prevention of burnout is a far better option that remedial treatment. Therapists should check in with themselves about their current functioning to avoid the "slippery slope" of burnout. Ideally, therapists will learn to apply their training in assessment and response to patients' needs and difficulties to themselves (Pelling & Burton, 2019). Key to this is frequent reflection, checking in regarding own mood and well-being, and noticing changes to key areas of functioning such as sleep, appetite, energy levels, engagement with friends and leisure activities, and negative symptoms such as irritability and flat mood.

It is no coincidence that many of the factors associated with burnout overlap with depressive symptoms. This can make it all the harder for therapists to identify their experience as burnout, depression, or perhaps reflective of another condition.

Symptoms of burnout for therapists may include:

- "Clock-watching" during a session (feeling time in the session with patients is going slowly, or willing time to pass more swiftly)
- Negative feelings towards patients, including resentment and anger
- Compassion fatigue
- Social isolation, and withdrawal from friends and family
- Poor nutrition or changes in diet
- Increased use of or dependence on alcohol or other drugs
- Poor sleep hygiene or changes to sleep
- Anhedonia (disinterest in usual leisure activities)

Therapists must be cognisant of their own needs and work towards alignment of these in their professional life. For me, a non-negotiable is a comfortable consulting room with natural light and windows that can be opened to allow for fresh air. (A surprising number of consulting rooms do not have these features!) Knowing that my mood and well-being are impacted by a lack of access to these, I ensure to prioritise these aspects in my professional practice.

It can be difficult to detect the slow slide into burnout. When recognised, it is important that the therapist does not carry on regardless. Burnout is never resolved by ignoring exhaustion. The only solution is proper rest and recuperation.

At times, therapists may need to decline referrals from patients whose concerns are similar to their own (Hackney & Cormier, 2012). Therapists are not immune to life crises or personal difficulties (Adams, 2024). Clear personal and clinical judgement is needed to decide if patients presenting with challenges similar to their own – such as relationship problems, infertility, parenting concerns, and substance or alcohol dependence – can be managed and treated without raising problematic issues around transference and countertransference. Sometimes the therapist will already be engaged in treatment with a patient when the events of their own parallel that of their patient. At these times, close supervision and consideration of countertransference is essential. It may be necessary to refer the patient to another therapist.

No therapist is obliged to accept every referral or see every patient. Nor is the therapist required to give a reason to prospective patients about their inability to accept a referral; it is sufficient to say, "I am not able to accept your referral at this time". Providing onward information about other suitable therapists who may be able to accept the referral is usually appreciated by the patient, but the therapist is not obliged to offer this.

Therapists often have personality features of perfectionism and are keen to please others and obtain approval; these can be adaptive characteristics in the helping professions and is associated with empathy and kind responses, making patients feel heard and understood. However, these personality features can also lead therapists to battle through personal difficulties without seeking assistance or taking stock of the impact on their professional work with patients. Therapists must be mindful of not falling into a "saviour complex", whereby the therapist has a need or compulsion to save others. The therapist overestimates their role in a patient's life, or contribution to a patient's well-being. The work of a therapist is important, but no therapist is indispensable, and any one therapist should never be the only source of assistance or care for any one patient.

Therapists need to be mindful of putting their own needs second to patients. Engage in hobbies, take leave, plan vacations, spend time with your family and friends. The analogy of parents needing to place an oxygen mask on themselves before fitting it on their children also holds true for therapists and their patients – a therapist experiencing burnout may be unhelpful and, in some cases, dangerous to the well-being of patients. My experience of telling patients of upcoming leave has been overwhelmingly positive; most patients understand that therapists – like all people – need to take a break from time to time. A therapist should never feel that they can never take leave from work. This dynamic must sometimes be managed differently with patients who exhibit borderline or dependent personality traits. For these patients, for whom a separation from their therapist may trigger responses of abandonment or distress, it may be beneficial to provide more notice of leave, develop a safety plan, or provide details of an alternate therapist to work with or contact during leave. It can also provide an opportunity for the therapist and patient to work through feelings such as abandonment, separation anxiety, and dependence (McWilliams, 1999).

Vicarious traumatisation

The practice of therapy is demanding. In comparison to other occupations or some other helping professions, therapists are exposed to a disproportionate amount of vicarious trauma. Vicarious traumatisation can occur from repeated exposure to hearing others' distressing experiences. This "traumatic contagion" can often be cumulative; rather than becoming inured to hearing others' recall of distressing experiences, research consistently shows a slow degradation of well-being over time (Clark et al., 2022; Cozolino, 2004). Repeated exposure to people who have had negative or traumatic experiences takes a slow but steady toll on therapists. Similar to burnout, all therapists are likely to experience vicarious traumatisation at some stage of their career, although it may go unrecognised or be assumed to be caused by other factors, such as workload or external life events.

Compassion fatigue can result from vicarious traumatisation. This is the antithesis of the necessary qualities of a therapist. This slow obliteration of the capacity to feel and express empathy for others is experienced to an extent by most therapists at some career stage. Often it coincides with difficulties in the therapist's own personal life or psychosocial stress associated with family members or loved ones (Türkel et al., 2025).

The same strategies useful in managing burnout can also apply to managing vicarious traumatisation and compassion fatigue. These include managing caseload to include a variety of presentations, and therapists being cognisant of potential triggers for countertransference based on their own significant life events or history of trauma. This should be considered and used in conjunction with other forms of self-care.

Self-care

Most drivers who have undertaken a long road trip will be familiar with warning signs to the effect of "sleepy drivers die" and "only sleep cures fatigue". Analogous to this for therapists is the mantra that "only rest cures burnout". Resist the temptation of seeking to revitalise the professional self by throwing oneself further into work.

Therapists have an obligation to care for themselves, in order to be able to best care for others. Pathological caregiving and denial of one's own needs is not helpful and in some situations may become decidedly unhelpful. This does not mean that therapists will never experience their own difficulties related to mental health or well-being. In fact, therapists are obliged to be aware of their mental health and well-being and to take appropriate measures to ensure their own experiences or concerns around mental health do not negatively impact their capacity to provide care and treatment to patients. Therapists are most helpful when they maintain efforts around good psychological health and do not feel distracted or overwhelmed by their own personal problems.

In addition to supervision and personal therapy (see Chapter 10), ongoing self-care is an integral activity and ethical obligation for all therapists. Self-care must be pre-emptive and planned, rather than remedial or reactive.

Four main domains of self-care are relevant to therapists (Corey et al., 2024):

1. Physical:
   - Exercise (especially important to counteract the sedentary nature of therapy, in which many hours are spent sitting)
   - Nutrition
   - Sleep
   - Engaging in positive life experiences
2. Emotional:
   - Monitoring own mood and well-being
   - Zest, vitality, excitement
   - Maintaining a sense of inner tranquillity and peace
3. Relationship:
   - Social interaction
   - Friendship
   - Romantic and / or physical intimacy
4. Spiritual:
   - Connectedness to self and others
   - Sense of holistic well-being
   - Capacity to recognise and value things beyond material elements
   - May not necessitate affiliation with any religious group or organised belief system

Therapy-specific factors and strategies include:

- Monitoring workload and patient numbers / caseload size. Plan ahead to ensure you have capacity to offer appointments without being overrun or needing to offer appointments outside of your usual work hours.
- Being mindful of patients' presenting problems and stage of treatment. A variety of presentations and having patients at different stages of treatment (assessment, treatment, maintenance) can help stave off burnout.
- Consider your daily schedule, ensuring breaks for lunch and other activities that are not related to work.
- Schedule regular time away from work. Plan leave and vacation time well in advance.

Self-care strategies for therapists

No single self-care strategy will be effective all of the time. A toolbox never comprises just one tool. It is therefore useful to have several strategies to draw upon.

Three useful strategies for therapists are detailed here: (i) escaping the therapist self; (ii) engaging in "worry time"; and (iii) and identifying areas of over-evaluation and opportunity for change.

A friend once remarked that she often forgot I was a psychologist, commenting on my apparent capacity to converse about topics unrelated to therapy and my tendency to "not take life too seriously". I thought this to be a terrific compliment; I have long believed the best self-care for therapists is to ensure periods of disengagement with therapy and all things therapy-related. First, an individual consumed with any one topic makes for a boring conversationalist. Second, the fastest way to burnout is a lack of diversity in life. In keeping with my need to occasionally disconnect from all things related to work, I sometimes choose to not disclose my vocation at social events or in circumstances such as sitting next to a stranger on an aeroplane. Experience tells me that in these situations, it is often inevitable that casual conversation will turn to self-disclosure from others around their own or others' mental health experiences.

To this end, it is beneficial for therapists to devote a good chunk of their life to activities that have nothing to do with therapy. If all you have is a hammer, then everything looks like a nail; in other words, if you think about all things in therapy terms, then you risk your view of the world becoming a pathologised place. Sometimes, the best thing a therapist can do for their own well-being is to look at life through a non-therapeutic lens. Patients and all their concerns will still be there when therapists return from their mental sojourn. A well-rested and revitalised therapist is able to offer patients optimal treatment.

"Worry time" is an excellent strategy for therapists prone to excessive rumination about patients outside of work hours. This is a paradoxical intervention of sorts; the therapist focuses on all patient and work-related matters for a set period of time (perhaps 15 minutes). When thoughts occur outside of this time, the therapist gently reminds themselves to hold over the thoughts until the next allocated "worry time". This strategy can also be useful for any person who finds themselves ruminating about work or a specific topic. If the rumination is leading to endless conversation (usually with a spouse or family member), the recipient of the information is encouraged to acknowledge the thought but point out that the conversation matter can be held over until the next allocated "worry time". This is a remarkably simple but effective intervention.

Last, therapists who have difficulties around their own self-care often over-evaluate the importance of work, leading to under-evaluation of other activities in life. This is then associated with problems around self-care, as work is prioritised and becomes a defining feature of their personality.

The following activity is adapted from Fairburn's (2008) seminal work with eating disorder patients. Similar to therapists who obsess about work or over-evaluate its importance, eating disorder patients often over-evaluate factors associated with eating, including food intake, restriction, weight, and shape. Patients are encouraged to construct two "pie charts": first, the components of their current thinking, and second, an idea of how things could be in the future. This proves a powerful exercise, especially when the completed pie charts are viewed concurrently. The exercise alerts the patient to the discrepancy between their actual and ideal lives. A further useful step to this exercise is to list ways in which a move from the actual to the ideal can be achieved. This may include joining a social group, investigating a hobby, or balancing unhelpful activities such as excessive social media reading fiction or non-fiction books.

This activity, as depicted in Figure 8.1, can be readily adapted to other clinical patients outside of the eating disorder population, and, more pertinently, to therapists.

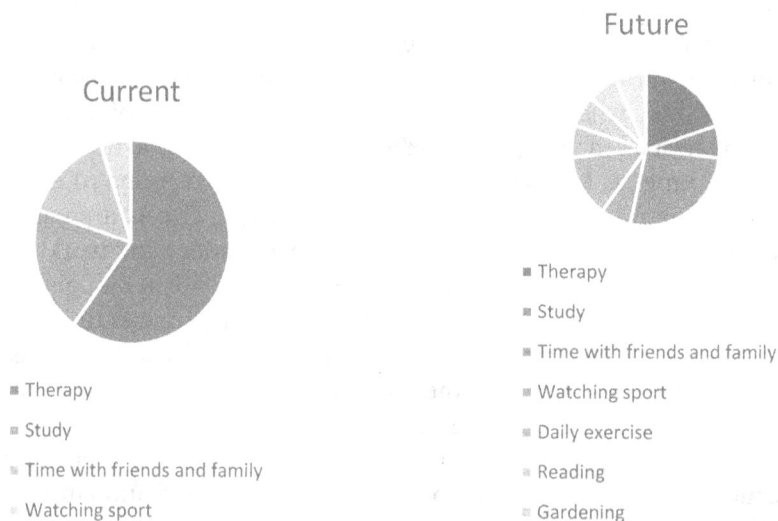

Current

Future

- Therapy
- Study
- Time with friends and family
- Watching sport

- Therapy
- Study
- Time with friends and family
- Watching sport
- Daily exercise
- Reading
- Gardening

Figure 8.1 Pie graph activity, adapted from Fairburn (2008).

Self-care and the activities related to it will look different for each therapist. My own self-care usually comprises a combination of yoga, walking, listening to a podcast (not related to therapy or true-crime; I avoid content that may prompt think about a formulation or worry about another person's well-being), reading fiction or non-fiction (again, nothing work-related), writing, walking, gardening, spending time with my children, and dinners or evenings out with friends. I am part of formal groups for both reading and writing; these maintain accountability in these activities and provide the added benefit of socialising with people who are not therapists. Others' self-care activities may include watching a television programme, going to the cinema, cooking, watching or participating in sport, building or maintenance tasks, or travel.

Summary

- Transference is the process by which a patient projects onto their therapist past feelings, experiences, or attitudes.
- Related to transference is the psychological phenomena of countertransference. This is the process by which a therapist projects onto their patient past feelings, experience, or attitudes.
- The psychological phenomena of transference and countertransference are often poorly understood by trainee and early-career therapists, leading to confusion and misapplication in clinical work.
- Recognising and managing transference and countertransference is an important element of relational therapeutic modalities. Transference and countertransference are primarily the remit of psychoanalytic and psychodynamic therapies; however, their importance and application to other therapeutic modalities is becoming more widely understood and appreciated.
- Therapist burnout can be a consequence of lack of attention to or lack of understanding around transference and countertransference. Burnout may also be precipitated by vicarious traumatisation, ill health, or personal crises.
- Burnout is a slow and insidious process by which the therapist reaches a state of exhaustion.
- Self-care is key to therapists' remaining in a state of professional competence. It is an ongoing process, rather than an end point.
- Strategies to promote self-care include managing workload and caseload, balancing work with leisure activities, and engaging in supervision and personal therapy.

Reference list

Adams, M. (2024). *The myth of the untroubled therapist* (2nd ed.). Routledge.

Barnett, J. E., Zimmerman, J., & Walfish, S. (2014). *The ethics of private practice: A practical guide for mental health clinicians.* Oxford University Press.

Berman, J. (2019). *Writing the talking cure: Irvin D. Yalom and the literature of psychotherapy.* State University of New York.

Clark, P., Holden, C., Russell, M., & Downs, H. (2022). The imposter phenomenon in mental health professionals: Relationships among compassion fatigue, burnout, and compassion satisfaction. *Contemporary Family Therapy, 44,* 185–197. https://doi.org/10.1007/s10591-021-09580-y

Corey, G., Corey, M. S., & Corey, C. (2024). *Issues & ethics in the helping professions* (11th ed.). Cengage.

Cozolino, L. (2004). *The making of a therapist.* Norton.

DeYoung, P. A. (2022). *Understanding and treating chronic shame: Healing right brain relational trauma.* Routledge.

Fairburn, C. G. (2008). *Cognitive behavior therapy and eating disorders.* Guilford Press.

Gabbard, G. O. (2005). *Psychodynamic psychiatry in clinical practice* (4th ed.). American Psychiatric Publications.

Hackney, H. L., & Cormier, S. (2012). *The professional counselor: A process guide to helping* (7th ed.). Pearson.

Jung, C. G. (1946). *The psychology of the transference.* Princeton University Press.

McWilliams, N. (1999). *Psychoanalytical case formulation.* Guilford Press.

Orange, D. (1995). *Emotional understanding: Studies in psychoanalytic epistemology.* Guilford Press.

Pelling, N., & Burton, L. J. (Eds.). (2019). *Elements of ethical practice: Applied psychology ethics in Australia.* Routledge.

Pocock, D. (2006). Six things worth understanding about psychoanalytic psychotherapy. *Journal of Family Therapy, 28*(4), 352–369. https://doi.org/10.1111/j.1467-6427.2006.00357.x

Türkel, N. N., Başaran, A. S., Gazey, H., & Ertek, İ. E. (2025). The imposter phenomenon in psychiatrists: Relationships among compassion fatigue, burnout, and maladaptive perfectionism. *BMC Psychiatry, 25*(1), 30. https://doi.org/10.1186/s12888-025-06470-7

Yalom, I. D. (1989). *Love's executioner and other tales of psychotherapy.* Basic Books.

Yalom, I. D. (2009). *The gift of therapy: Reflections on being a therapist.* Harper Perennial.

Ethical and professional decision-making for therapists

9

Knowledge and application of ethics is a core area of competence for all therapists. Practising in a professional manner and with good faith is imperative to provide for the safety of patients. In turn, practising in a way that is consistent with ethical principles also safeguards therapists against providing treatment that is inappropriate, unethical, or potentially harmful.

Knowledge of ethics receives significant coverage in all therapy training courses. This speaks to the importance of ethical conduct for all therapists. Through studies and training, most therapists are familiar with ethical principles and codes of conduct or ethical guidelines relevant to clinical practice. Many therapists can apply these to ethical scenarios and can confidently "solve" the dilemmas presented in hypothetical case studies and clinical vignettes. However, real-life scenarios are inherently more nuanced and complex. Hence, for many trainee and early-career therapists, applying decision-making to real-life ethical dilemmas can seem daunting. In the face of a "real" ethical dilemma, it can be tempting for novice therapists to fall back onto their personal decision-making skills (including intuition, gut instinct, and personal judgement). Instead, professional skills and knowledge around ethics and professional behaviour should be employed.

"There are thousands of ethical dilemmas that can take place. One-on-one therapy means that the therapist can be vulnerable too. Putting the needs of the client is paramount, but ensure you cover yourself at the same time!"

DOI: 10.4324/9781003533030-9

Ethical dilemmas

Ethical dilemmas occur when one or more ethical principles has been breached or is at risk of being breached. Inherent to an ethical dilemma is the multitude of choices that may be employed to resolve the dilemma. For therapists, common ethical dilemmas include concerns around confidentiality, dual roles or multiple relationships, and working with patients who present with risk of harm to self or others.

The terms "professional issue" or "professional dilemma" are sometimes used interchangeably with "ethical dilemma". While the two are conceptually similar, professional issues are typically associated with problems related to professional conduct, such as business practices and interactions with patients that occur outside the consulting room. Professional issues or professional dilemmas are not usually directly relevant to treatment. It is possible to act ethically while not maintaining professionalism. For example, not returning a patient's phone call in a timely manner or wearing casual clothes to work both represent professional issues, but they do not necessarily indicate unethical behaviour. Conversely, it is possible (but less likely) to behave unethically while maintaining a professional standard.

The decision-making models presented in this chapter are typically applied to ethical dilemmas but can also be applied to professional issues.

Ethical decision-making

Therapy is replete with ethical dilemmas. These may include individual concerns of a relatively small scale, such as the decision-making of a therapist about whether to accept a referral when a multiple relationship with the patient may occur, or whether to charge a cash-strapped patient a cancellation fee. On a broader scale, the therapy professions are concerned with social issues, such as debates around the acceptability of euthanasia, the morals of capital punishment, or decision-making around assisted fertility.

Identifying whether an issue is, in fact, an ethical dilemma, can present an initial challenge. This can be especially true for novice therapists who are attempting to balance the learning or mastery of therapy skills with consideration of ethical issues.

The following strategies and questions may help therapists to consider the nature of the problem, and to clarify whether the concern is in fact an ethical dilemma (Shaw et al., 2013):

- Take another perspective on the problem:
  - Ask yourself, "Would I feel comfortable if my colleagues knew about this situation?"

- Reflect on change to behaviour:
  - "Have I changed my usual professional standards?"
  - "Have I increased my self-disclosure, or am I experiencing increased rumination after sessions with this patient?"
  - "How do I feel in the room with this patient? Do I experience any unease or discomfort?"
- Ascertain legal implications:
  - "Is this a legal problem rather than an ethical dilemma?"
  - "Are there relevant laws or legislation relevant here?"
- Reflect on implications of the ethical dilemma and its management:
  - "Could this dilemma have been prevented?"

Ethical decision-making is a skill that requires practice. The following tips provide a quick reference for key points to consider when faced with an ethical dilemma:

- Decide whether the problem is, in fact, an ethical dilemma.
- Identify relevant ethical principles.
- Zoom out on the problem, rather than focus on the minutiae of a patient's presentation or details of their experience.
- Consult codes of conduct and other professional documents, as relevant.
- Apply an ethical decision-making model to all ethical dilemmas.
- Do not rush the decision-making process. Resist pressure from others and the self to reach a fast resolution.
- Engage in extra supervision, as necessary. This may include primary supervision, peer supervision, and additional supervision with a therapist who has expertise and experience relevant to the ethical dilemma.
- Obtain legal advice and/or guidance from your professional association, if appropriate.
- Document all stages of the decision-making process, including the outcome and the application of the outcome.

Ethical principles

Trainee and early-career therapists often become weighed down in the minutiae of a patient's story. This can make it difficult to see the woods for the trees. This myopic view can shape the therapist's decision-making and may negatively impact the therapist's capacity to manage and resolve an ethical dilemma.

Therapists need to be mindful of being caught up in superfluous details. It is crucial for therapists to have the capacity to provide a succinct overview of the ethical dilemma under consideration, rather than become caught up in a "he said, she said" recall of events. Here, clinical judgment and the use of professional rather than informal language is essential to ensure focus on relevant information. Zooming out on a problem can provide the clarity needed to objectively judge an ethical dilemma and make informed decisions around the best course of action.

Knowledge of ethical principles is imperative. These provide broad "umbrella terms" that can be applied to communicate the relevant themes and issues inherent to the ethical dilemma. Referring to ethical principles reduces unnecessary information and hence informs efficient and effective decision-making. Sound knowledge of ethical principles and their application provide an essential foundation to understanding ethical dilemmas. It is the responsibility of each therapist to be familiar with the ethical principles relevant to their profession.

The ethical principles listed in Table 9.1 are typically considered relevant to therapy and other helping professions. The principles are integrated

Table 9.1 Key ethical principles for decision-making.

Autonomy	Respect for patients' independence and self-determination. The principle of autonomy guides therapists to support patients making their own decisions and acting in accordance with their own values. The application of autonomy depends on the therapist's judgement of the patient being able to make sound and rational decisions; some patients, such as children and individuals with mental impairment, are not able to make autonomous decisions.
Justice	Therapists promote fairness, impartiality, and equity in their treatment of patients.
Beneficence	Therapists strive to practise in a manner that is beneficial to patients. Therapists are mindful of patients' welfare, and work in a way that supports and encourages their well-being. This encompasses "doing good", but also extends to preventing harm, if necessary.
Fidelity	Therapists are loyal and faithful in their practice and work. They honour commitments, meet obligations, and are true to promises made. Fidelity is establishing and maintaining trust between therapist and patient, and is hence integral to a good therapeutic relationship.
Non-maleficence	Therapists are careful to not cause harm to patients. This includes not inflicting intentional harm and extends to not engaging in actions that risk harming patients or other people.

into codes of conduct and ethical codes, hence providing a foundation for expectations around professional behaviour and clinical practice (Forester-Miller & Davis, 1995).

No code of conduct or code of ethics provides answers to specific ethical dilemmas. In lieu of a "blueprint" to resolve ethical dilemmas, the codes reflect a set of principles that can be applied to specific queries and used to provide guidance on moral problems. Such codes reflect the collective wisdom of the profession, providing an indication of the prevailing professional stance and perspectives on important ethical issues (Corey et al., 2024; Cozolino, 2004).

With regards to ethics, there is generally "nothing new under the sun", in that existing principles and guidelines can be applied to modern issues. In this sense, codes of conduct or ethical guidelines may not yet reflect specific novel issues experienced by therapists. For example, the ethical considerations around processing online credit card payments for patients is a relatively new issue. However, concerns around this process may be considered under pre-existing guidelines related to financial arrangements, and may be covered under the ethical principle of *fidelity* (i.e., therapists maintain honesty and fairness in financial dealings). Novice therapists can take some comfort in this – while details may differ, successive generations of therapists have experienced similar ethical dilemmas. The collective knowledge and experience of these therapists are reflected within the codes of conduct and ethical guidelines.

Challenges associated with decision-making

Applying appropriate decision-making and resolving ethical dilemmas can be particularly challenging for trainee and early-career therapists. With the primary remit of novice therapists being acquiring knowledge and mastering skills, therapists at these career stages can understandably feel overwhelmed or blindsided by ethical dilemmas. The lurch of switching gears from therapy skills to ethical decision-making can feel difficult; however, in reality these often co-exist, and therapists must become adept at balancing both.

Most often, trainee and early-career therapists exhibit high standards of professional behaviour and demonstrate a strong awareness of their responsibility to practise in an ethical manner. Many novice therapists are hypervigilant about any professional behaviour that may result in being brought to the attention of a professional body or licensing board, or, even worse, engaging in any conduct that may result in disciplinary action

(Cozolino, 2004). This may be a reflection of personality characteristics of perfectionism, or it may be an outcome of training in which ethics and professional standards are a strong focus of learning.

Ethical dilemmas experienced by therapists are not typically of a salacious nature, such as those including sexual relationships between therapists and patients. The dilemmas most commonly experienced by therapists are generally less newsworthy and do not typically reach the media or garner the public's attention. Common ethical dilemmas include the following (Barnett et al., 2014; Frankcom et al., 2016):

- Referral and intake issues (deciding appropriateness of referral, referral triage, waitlist management, ensuring informed consent)
- Confidentiality breaches (unauthorised sharing of patients' private information, therapists' communication with parents of child and adolescent patients)
- Practising outside of one's scope of competence, knowledge, or training
- Persisting with treatment in the absence of improvement in the patient's condition
- Ensuring appropriate continuity of care following termination of treatment

Models of decision-making

Professional decision-making differs from the problem-solving strategies used for personal problems. A conversation with a friend or family member may be useful for personal concerns. In these situations, information is shared freely, and people may be encouraged to trust their intuition about a problem, or to "follow their gut". Professional decision-making, however, is driven by ethical principles, clinical judgment, and professional standards.

"Ethical decision making is a teachable skill."

To this end, therapists are advised to consult a decision-making model to resolve ethical dilemmas. Several models are popular among therapists, and more broadly within the helping professions. Forester-Miller and Davis (1995) offer a seven-step model that integrates key features of several well-known ethical-decision-making theories, emphasising parts of each model most relevant to counsellors. Similar eight- and nine-step models have been proposed by Kämpf (2009) and Koocher and Keith-Spiegel (2016), respectively.

While each model has unique features, common to all is the series of steps that enable the therapist to operationalise and understand the ethical dilemma, apply ethical principles, propose possible solutions, weigh the advantages and disadvantages of each proposed solution, implement the solution, and then evaluate its efficacy.

Also inherent to all decision-making models is documentation and record-keeping. This is an essential stage of ethical decision-making. Therapists cannot always guarantee the outcome of decision-making around an ethical dilemma, but they can ensure their notes and records of the patient, the ethical dilemma, and the decision-making process are complete and current. These records are especially crucial in the instance of a complaint being brought against a therapist; it is important to be able to demonstrate the knowledge and reasoning that informed the therapist's decision-making process relevant to the complaint. Disciplinary boards are interested in the decision-making process, not simply the outcome. This recognises the nuance and complexity of ethical dilemmas.

"Not just the decision that is made, but how the decision is made. If unsure, use the support of colleagues to problem-solve or act as devil's advocate."

Worked example of ethical decision-making

A worked example of an ethical dilemma is detailed here. In this hypothetical case, the therapist was referred to mandated supervision by a regulatory body, following a complaint by a colleague regarding concerns about their clinical practice.

This case exemplifies the merit of using a structured decision-making framework to work through ethical dilemmas. While always imperative, this process is particularly useful when working with patients with complex presentations, or those who present with unusual or novel presentations.

Background information

Sarah is an early-career therapist who has recently commenced work in a medium-sized private practice. In this role, she practises under the supervision of the directors of the clinic and also obtains external supervision on a monthly basis.

Sarah recently commenced therapy sessions with Tate, a 30-year-old man referred to treatment as a part of a court order. Mandated therapy sessions were ordered as part of Tate's conviction for indecent public behaviour. Tate had accessed pornographic material on his smartphone while a passenger on a metropolitan train. Tate was wearing headphones; however, these were not paired with his smartphone, and as such the sound associated with the pornographic video was audible to other passengers.

Sarah did not have previous experience in working with forensic patients or other patients engaging in court-mandated treatment; however, the clinic directors encouraged Sarah to accept the referral. They cited reasons of broadening her clinical experience, financial benefit to the clinic and to Sarah, and the need for Sarah to establish and build her case load and reputation. The clinic directors also expressed a desire to maintain a good business relationship with the referrer, who was known to provide a steady stream of referrals to the clinic.

Tate presented in casual dress. He was well groomed, clean-shaven, with neatly cropped hair. No tattoos or other distinguishing features were noted. Tate was affable and engaged well in initial and subsequent therapy sessions. He was punctual for each appointment. Mood was euthymic with congruent affect. Tate was talkative and occasionally difficult to contain; he often initiated discussion with little prompt required from Sarah. Sessions often ran over time, with Tate raising important points in the last few minutes of session.

Tate explained the background of the conviction and court order to Sarah. Without prompting, he admitted the incident of indecent behaviour had occurred; however, he stated he was unaware that other passengers in the train carriage could see pornographic material or hear the associated audio. He reported being "devastated" to have potentially caused offence or made others feel uncomfortable, and hence he had not opposed the conviction despite encouragement from his lawyer to enter a plea of no guilt.

Again without prompting, Tate acknowledged his pornography use to be problematic. He stated that he watched pornography for up to five hours per day, usually accessing it at home but increasingly in public places such as on public transport, during walks around his neighbourhood, and while shopping at places such as the supermarket or department store. Tate experienced insomnia as a consequence of the pornography addiction. He was becoming socially isolated from friends, and he declared no interest in dating. Tate reported a lack of interest in his usual leisure activities, including watching sport and reading sci-fi novels.

Tate stated that he was keen to engage in therapy sessions to "finally get some help". He expressed hoped that the court-mandated sessions could be used to treat his pornography addiction.

During the third therapy session, Tate told Sarah of a therapeutic intervention he had read about on an online forum. The treatment involved "exposure therapy", during which the patient and therapist watched pornography together. Tate detailed that the aim of the "exposure therapy" was for the therapist to help the patient identify thoughts and feelings that occurred while watching pornography. Tate said he was keen to start on this treatment as soon as possible. He proposed watching two 10-minute pornographic videos each session, followed by a discussion of his thoughts and feelings about the content, commencing with next week's session.

Sarah was familiar with "exposure therapy" for anxiety disorders (i.e., treatment of conditions such as PTSD and phobias), but had not heard of this as a specific treatment for pornography addiction.

Tate's proposition for treatment represented an ethical dilemma for Sarah. She is unsure of how to continue with treatment sessions. At the encouragement of her supervisor, Sarah applied a decision-making model to the ethical dilemma.

Decision-making model

Sarah selected the nine-step ethical decision-making model proposed by Koocher and Keith-Spiegel (2016). She was familiar with this model through an ethics unit undertaken at University, and hence had a good understanding of the steps involved.

Step 1: Determine whether the matter is an ethical one

In determining whether concerns related to Tate's treatment were indeed an ethical matter, Sarah first identified the relevant ethical principles – autonomy, beneficence, and fidelity.

Autonomy, defined as the patient's right to make decisions about their own treatment, is relevant, as Tate presented as insightful, well-informed, and keen to engage in treatment. *Beneficence*, defined as the therapist's obligation to "do good" and promote well-being, was also important to consider. *Fidelity*, defined in this context as honesty and integrity, is relevant, as Sarah is unsure about the credibility and evidence base for the treatment proposed by Tate.

Step 2: Consult available guidelines that might apply to a specific identification and possible mechanism for resolution

Sarah consulted relevant guidelines, including the relevant Code of Conduct for her profession. The document provided guidance rather than clear directives regarding resolving this specific ethical dilemma. In particular, Sarah focused on information related to:

- Working within one's scope of competence
- Recognising the patient's right to make decisions about treatment
- Providing treatment consistent with evidence-based practice
- Providing an environment in which the patient feels safe and supported
- Never establishing a sexual relationship with patients
- Recognising and taking steps to minimise risk to the therapist
- Seeking advice from an experienced clinician and/or supervisor, where appropriate

Step 3: Consider, as best as possible, all sources that might influence the decision you will make

In addition to relevant guidelines and documents, other factors that might influence the decision relevant to Tate's treatment were considered. This included exploration of personal factors. A comprehensive review of relevant literature was also undertaken.

First, Sarah considered personal factors that might influence her decision. This focused on her own views about pornography and its use. Sarah concluded that her views regarding pornography were generally neutral, in that she did not hold negative assumptions about its use or those who view it. Sarah also noted that she was not particularly familiar with pornography, including the many genres of pornography and the ways in which pornography may be accessed and used.

"We all have blind-spots. Be open to supervision, your own therapy, and be inquisitive and vulnerable about where your blind spots and biases might lie."

Second, Sarah conducted a comprehensive literature review. Having identified that she did not have a great deal of knowledge about pornography,

Sarah investigated the research literature regarding pornography addiction. Through her initial literature search, Sarah realised she would need to re-familiarise herself with general research around addiction, in addition to literature more specific to pornography addiction.

First, Sarah consulted broader information regarding addiction. In particular, she found it helpful to revisit course content and prescribed and suggested readings regarding paraphilic disorders and addiction from her recently completed training (Herring, 2001; Nichols, 2006). Next, Sarah identified articles about the psychological aspects of pornography use and the aetiology (i.e., causes) of pornography addiction. This included recent meta-analyses (Antons et al., 2022; Wright et al., 2016). These readings informed her general understanding of the topic, including considering Tate's behaviour as an impulse-control condition, a compulsive behaviour, or, potentially, a paraphilia-related disorder (Antons et al., 2022).

Sarah also searched for information specific to exposure therapy for pornography addiction. She was unable to identify any research findings or broader academic literature around this. This absence of academic attention led Sarah to consider that exposure therapy was not an evidence-based treatment for pornography addiction. Within the literature, psychotherapy and/or CBT was identified as the most frequent treatment intervention. Art therapy, a 12-step approach, and psychopharmacological therapy were also cited as treatments (Antons et al., 2022). Sarah could not locate any published literature to support the notion that a therapist participating in exposure therapy with a patient represented an evidence-based treatment for pornography addiction.

Step 4: Consult with others

Sarah consulted several colleagues, including her supervisor. Her supervisor also suggested seeking specialised supervision with an external supervisor, as they noted their own lack of experience and current knowledge in the field of addiction and pornography addiction.

Sarah also discussed Tate's case within her peer supervision group. Given the nature of the query related to pornography, Sarah initially felt apprehensive about sharing the details of the case. However, Sarah was buoyed by the professionalism and support of her peers, who demonstrated empathy and understanding.

In some cases related to ethical dilemmas, it may also be necessary to obtain guidance or advice beyond colleagues and supervisors. Members of professional associations may also be able to access information from advisory boards, which are usually staffed by senior clinicians with experience in clinical work and ethical decision-making.

---

*"Being a member of a professional organisation
has also helped me many times!"*

Step 5: Evaluate the rights, responsibilities, and vulnerabilities of all affected parties

Affected parties included Tate and Sarah. Members of the public were also considered affected parties, as they had been exposed to pornography and there was a risk of this occurring again.

As a patient, Tate has the right to autonomy in the selection of and participation in treatment.

Sarah identified both herself and the members of the public as vulnerable. Sarah considered that Tate may be manipulating her into viewing pornography. In considering members of the public, Sarah thought of their right to safety when in public places, and she also considered the presence of children in public places, including trains and other forms of transport.

Sarah identified herself as responsible for providing evidence-based treatment. Her role as Tate's therapist was to promote his well-being, but also to protect her own well-being. Sarah noted concerns regarding her own discomfort around the proposed exposure therapy, which would include Sarah watching pornography with Tate.

Step 6: Generate alternative decisions

Koocher and Keith-Spiegel (2016) state that all options should be considered at this stage of the decision-making process, regardless of the apparent feasibility of each. Nothing is disregarded prior to thorough consideration of its viability. This may result in the inclusion of options initially deemed too risky, costly, or otherwise unlikely for extraneous reasons. After all factors are weighed and considered, a different perspective may be gained regarding those options initially deemed unfavourable.

Option A: Proceed with exposure therapy, as proposed by Tate.
Option B: Propose a different form of treatment.
Option C: Do not commence any treatment with Tate.

Table 9.2 Benefits and disadvantages of decision outcomes.

	Benefits	Disadvantages
Option A: Process with exposure therapy, as proposed by Tate	• Therapeutic benefit with Tate will not be negatively impacted. • Tate's autonomy is respected.	• No evidence base for exposure therapy for pornography addiction. • Sarah's discomfort at engaging in treatment.
Option B: Propose a different form of treatment	• Safeguards Sarah from potential professional and personal discomfort and harm. • Fulfils Sarah's ethical obligation to provide evidence-based treatment. • The proven efficacy of an evidence-based treatment provides Tate with the best chance of an optimal treatment outcome.	• Tate may not be willing to engage with a different form of treatment. • Sarah is not specifically trained in treatment for addiction. Further training and knowledge would be required, together with specific supervision with a therapist with expertise and experience in treatment of pornography addiction.
Option C: Do not commence any treatment with Tate	• Sarah satisfies her ethical obligations of doing no harm.	• If no treatment options are provided by Sarah, Tate may not receive any treatment at all. • Sarah learns nothing further about pornography addiction and its treatment, and therefore will not have knowledge for future similar referrals.

Step 7: Enumerate the consequences of making each decision

See Table 9.2 for an examination of the benefits and disadvantages of the proposed options.

Step 8: Make the decision

The decision was reached to propose a different form of treatment. This decision was supported by Sarah's access to specialised supervision provided by a therapist with expertise and experience in the field of pornography addiction. At the suggestion of this supervisor, Sarah also enrolled in further training specific to pornography addiction. She also expanded upon her literature search in order to plan assessment and treatment suitable for Tate's presentation.

Step 9: Implement the decision

The decision was communicated to Tate in the next therapy session. As a part of informed consent, Sarah explained to Tate that he was free to decline the treatment options and seek treatment with another therapist.

Tate agreed to participate in the proposed treatment. Sarah provided an overview of evidence-based therapy for pornography addiction.

Last, the decision was documented in Tate's file. Sarah reviewed the decision with her supervisor and also provided a follow-up to her peer supervision group.

Ethical dilemmas involving other therapists

Observing another therapist practising in an unethical or unprofessional manner can be both surprising and disappointing. This can be especially true for novice therapists, who generally hold experienced therapists in high esteem.

Therapists hold a shared responsibility to ensure ethical behaviour and safeguard the public against untoward or unethical practice. Ignoring an ethical violation committed by a colleague is, in fact, an ethical violation. Junior status (in age or years of experience) does not preclude any therapist from this obligation.

Sometimes, current patients may raise concerns about a therapist with whom they have previously worked. Depending on the nature of the complaint, the therapist can encourage the patient to contact the relevant licensing body or registration board.

Concerns about others' professional and ethical behaviour can be managed using a step-by-step process. As shown in Figure 9.1, this process includes identifying the concern, and, if reasonable to do so, communicating the concern directly with the colleague. This acknowledges the professional standing of all involved and encourages the right of all parties to be fully informed at all stages of any complaint process. If the concern

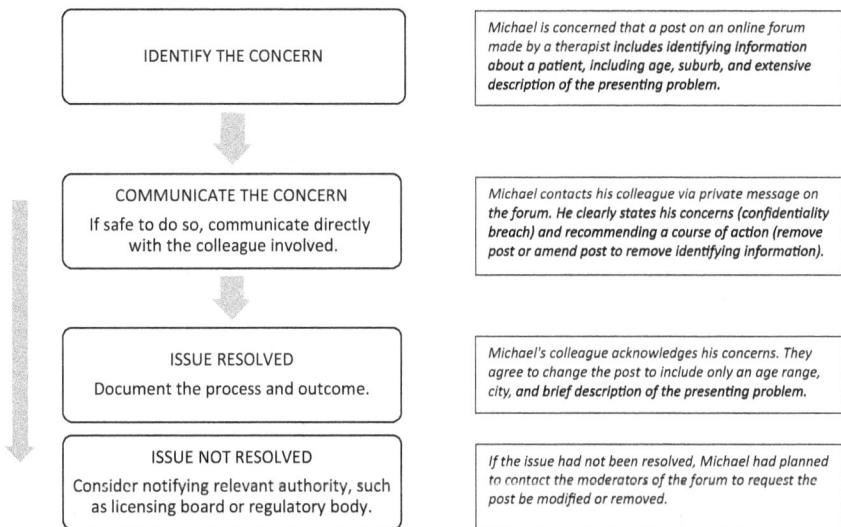

Figure 9.1 Managing concerns about others' professional or ethical behaviour.

is not resolved following this communication, the therapist may consider notifying the licensing board or other relevant authority.

As always, therapists should seek supervision to help guide decision-making around ethical dilemmas, including those related to other professionals' behaviour.

Summary

- Therapists often face ethical dilemmas. These can be especially challenging for novice therapists, who are balancing the mastery of therapy skills with ethical considerations and ethical decision-making.
- Ethical dilemmas occur when an ethical principle has been breached or is at risk of being breached, or when one or more ethical principles are in conflict.
- Key ethical principles relevant to therapy include: autonomy, justice, beneficence, fidelity, and non-maleficence.
- Documents, including codes of conduct and ethical guidelines, provide moral guidance for therapists. However, there is no "blueprint" to resolve ethical dilemmas, nor are there specific answers to particular ethical dilemmas.

- Decision-making models provide structure and guidance to resolve ethical dilemmas. Key steps within these models include: identifying the ethical dilemma, applying ethical principles, proposing possible solutions, and implementing the decision. Clear and contemporaneous documentation and record-keeping is important for all stages of the decision-making process.
- Therapists hold a shared responsibility to uphold ethical practice across the profession. To this end, therapists who notice others' behaviour to be unethical or unprofessional are obliged to take action.

Reference list

Antons, S., Engel, J., Briken, P., Krüger, T. H. C., Brand, M., & Stark, R. (2022). Treatments and interventions for compulsive sexual behavior disorder with a focus on problematic pornography use: A preregistered systematic review. *Journal of Behavioral Addictions*, 11(3), 643–666. https://doi.org/10.1556/2006.2022.00061

Barnett, J. E., Zimmerman, J., & Walfish, S. (2014). *The ethics of private practice: A practical guide for mental health clinicians*. Oxford University Press.

Corey, G., Corey, M. S., & Corey, C. (2024). *Issues & ethics in the helping professions* (11th ed.). Cengage.

Cozolino, L. (2004). *The making of a therapist*. Norton.

Forester-Miller, H., & Davis, T. E. (1995). *Practitioner's guide to ethical decision making*. American Counseling Association. https://www.counseling.org/docs/default-source/ethics/practioner-39-s-guide-to-ethical-decision-making.pdf

Frankcom, K., Stevens, B., & Watts, P. (2016). *Fit to practice*. Australian Academic Press.

Herring, B. (2001). Ethical guidelines in the treatment of compulsive sexual behavior. *Sexual Addiction & Compulsivity*, 8(1), 13–22. https://doi.org/10.1080/10720160127558

Kåmpf, A. (2009). *Confidentiality for mental health professional: A guide to ethical and legal principles*. Australian Academic Press.

Koocher, G. P., & Keith-Spiegel, P. (2016). *Ethics in psychology and the mental health professions: Standards and cases* (4th ed.). Oxford University Press.

Nichols, M. (2006). Psychotherapeutic issues with "kinky" clients: Clinical problems, yours and theirs. *Journal of Homosexuality*, 50(2–3), 281–300.

Shaw, E., Bancroft, H., Metzer, J., & Symons, M. (2013). Professional practice: How to make a sound ethical decision. *InPsych*, 35(6).

Wright, P. J., Tokunaga, R. S., & Kraus, A. (2016). A meta-analysis of pornography consumption and actual acts of sexual aggression in general population studies: Pornography and sexual aggression. *Journal of Communication*, 66(1), 183–205. https://doi.org/10.1111/jcom.12201

Supervision   **10**

"I am too busy seeing patients to make time for supervision."
"I don't have any challenging patients at the moment."
"I know what I am doing."
"I can't find a good supervisor."
"Supervision is expensive."
"A supervisor cannot teach me anything I do not already know."

Therapists often cite these reasons as justification for lack of engagement with supervision. There may be varying degrees of truth to each statement; however, none are sufficient to excuse participation in supervision. More likely, avoidance of supervision is informed by deep-seated yet unacknowledged concerns: insecurity, concerns about receiving feedback, fear of judgement, arrogance, and, for a small number of therapists, a truly narcissistic position in which the therapist believes they are superior to all others and therefore do not need oversight (McWilliams, 2011).

Behind all good therapy is good supervision. Every single therapist, whether in practice for two years or two decades, requires ongoing professional supervision. Therapy is not a career in which one can be self-sufficient; supervision is fundamental to therapists' practice being ethical and professional (Adams, 2024; Frankcom et al., 2016).

Supervision and its aims

Definitions of supervision vary across academic and clinical literature (Barnett et al., 2014). It is defined here as a reciprocal relationship during

DOI: 10.4324/9781003533030-10

which a more senior or experienced therapist offers training and oversight on legal, ethical, and professional issues.

The general aims of supervision include (Corey et al., 2024):

- Promoting supervisees' growth and development
- Protecting the welfare of patients
- Monitoring supervisees' performance
- Gate-keeping the profession (particularly in instances of concerns regarding competence or professional behaviour)
- Empowering the supervisee towards self-supervision

While essential across the entirety of a therapist's career trajectory, supervision is particularly important for trainee and early-career therapists. In recognition of this, supervision is typically mandated and embedded into training programmes. Close and frequent supervision in initial stages of training usually taper in frequency and intensity as the trainee works towards a more autonomous and independent practice.

Typically, supervision of trainees focuses heavily on skill development and the basic principles of "being in the room" with patients (see Chapter 2). Fundamental tasks such as note-taking and record-keeping are usually also included. Over time, supervision evolves to focus on more advanced concepts. This may include issues related to process (rather than content) of sessions, transference and countertransference, more complex diagnostic queries, and development of the therapist's identity and professional sense of self.

"Aspects of what we are told are hard to bear alone.
Good supervision, peer review, and reflective practice can
help ensure you tell stories about your work so you aren't
as alone with what you experience."

It is essential to document all participation in supervision. This includes logging hours and also keeping a record of the content of each supervision session. Most training organisations and professional bodies provide templates of logbooks and documents for supervision hours and supervision content, respectively. Record-keeping is usually a requirement for registration bodies or licensing boards, but it is also useful for future reference and provides a reminder of decision-making around clinical and ethical issues.

Types of supervision

As outlined in Table 10.1, therapists typically engage in several types of supervision. Ideally, a combination of these will be utilised to suit individual needs.

Individual supervision

Supervision is commonly thought of as a one-on-one relationship between a supervisor and supervisee, in which a more experienced therapist provides guidance and feedback to a novice or junior therapist.

The format of individual supervision will depend on the supervisee's stage of training, level of expertise, and years of clinical experience. Typically, supervision in initial stages of training is strongly informed by the supervisor. The structure of supervision will be led by the supervisor. As the trainee develops experience, they should be encouraged to contribute to shaping the structure and content of supervision. In this way, the supervisor models behaviour for the supervisee, thus shaping the supervisee's development and progress.

Table 10.1 Types of supervision.

Individual	One-on-one supervision between a therapist and a more senior or experienced therapist.
Group	A small group (4–5) of therapists engage in supervision facilitated by a more senior or experienced therapist.
Peer	Regular meetings of a small group of therapists, usually with similar levels of expertise and seniority. These are typically long-standing groups with permanent members.
Specialist	Ad-hoc supervision around a presentation or concern outside the scope of existing supervisor or supervisory relationship.
Self	The supervisee integrates and applies knowledge from supervision to their own practice, in the absence of direct input from a supervisor.
Remedial	Mandated by a professional body or licensing board, typically after an infringement or patient complaint.

> *"Therapists need access to reflective practice,*
> *peer review, and supervision."*

A number of strategies are essential to good supervision. As listed in Table 10.2, these overlap with many of the tasks inherent to good therapy, including agenda setting, structure, and feedback. It is also important for both the supervisor and supervisee to be aware of requirements around training and registration; for example, some programmes may require all notes and reports prepared by a trainee to be co-signed by a supervisor. Direct observation of the supervisee (usually via video recording) is also a standard requirement.

Table 10.2 Useful strategies for individual supervision.

Agenda setting	An agenda of items to be discussed should be tabled at the start of each supervision session. This is similar to the structure of a therapy session with patients. Initially this can be directed by the supervisor, with the supervisee encouraged to take increased responsibility for agenda setting over time.
	The benefits of prioritising items and allocating specific time to each is twofold: first, pertinent issues are covered; second, the skill of time management is demonstrated to the supervisee in a direct and observable way.
Observation of supervisee	Observation of supervisee during a patient session may be in-person but is most typically via review of video and/or audio recordings.
	Consulting rooms equipped with one-way mirrors can facilitate direct supervision. This provides an excellent opportunity for the supervisee to obtain real-time feedback from supervisors.
	Video and audio recordings provide for convenience and ease of supervisee observation. Informed consent from patients must be obtained before any video or audio recording. Appropriate storage and destruction of recordings must also be planned. For video recordings, note that the camera may be positioned to obscure the patient's face; the focus of supervision is usually on the supervisee, not their patient.
	A useful strategy for reviewing video and audio recordings involves supervisees selecting three sections for supervisors to review (noting that supervisors will not often have capacity or time to review full sessions). Sections of approximately five minutes can be chosen to demonstrate: (1) a skill of technique performed well; (2) an area that could be improved upon or about which the supervisee would like feedback; and (3) a query around formulation or diagnosis.

(Continued)

Table 10.2 (Continued)

Role play	The notion of participating in a "role play" usually elicits a collective groan from supervisees. Engaging in a role play (either as therapist or patient) can be daunting. It requires quick thinking and cognitive flexibility, placing the supervisee in a position of vulnerability. However, it represents an invaluable learning experience when conducted in a safe and secure supervisory relationship.
Process notes and case reports	Regular review of process notes and case reports is required for the supervisor to evaluate the supervisee's competence around written elements of therapy work. Supervision around notes and case reports may also include issues related to ethical and legal queries, such as when notes and reports are subpoenaed or requested by third parties. Feedback typically focuses on two areas: content and process. For content, feedback includes format, length of document, inclusion of essential information, being parsimonious with information, and writing in clinical rather than informal or expressive language. For process, supervision focuses on taking notes in session (type and amount), time management around case notes and reports, and rules and processes around storage and destruction of patient files.
Formulation	A formulation is a written synopsis of the therapist's informed ideas about the patient. It may include diagnosis but is moreover focused on the factors that contribute to the patient's current presentation. Known by the shorthand of the "four P's", a formulation includes predisposing, precipitating, perpetuating, and protective factors. The tasks around formulation can be modified to suit the supervisee's level of training and skill. Typically, a new trainee will be able to identify each of the "four P's" in isolation but will not yet be able to integrate these in a meaningful way. It is sufficient to list each factor separately, perhaps using a matrix or grid to organise the factors (noting that there is often overlap between factors). As the supervisee develops in understanding and skill, the supervisor can encourage the formulation to be written up in a longer and more sophisticated document. Completing a formulation for each patient is a valuable exercise. This activity promotes self-supervision and development of important clinical skills. Given time constraints, it is not usually possible to present a detailed formulation for each patient in supervision. The supervisee should be encouraged to present a diverse range of formulations that demonstrates their clinical skills and understanding.

Group supervision

Group supervision involves a small group (four to six therapists) who meet regularly to discuss clinical matters and case presentations. The group is facilitated by a more experienced or senior therapist. This type of supervision is often mandated as part of training.

In addition to discussion of clinical matters and patients, group supervision offers the chance to build relationships with colleagues and obtain a good social support system with therapists at similar levels of experience. Strong professional relationships and lifelong friendships are often borne out of supervision groups.

> *"Read widely and trawl through books and papers,*
> *both contemporary and those from the past. At first,*
> *reading might leave you bewildered. Don't stress. Read*
> *what makes most sense to you and talk about the ideas with*
> *your colleagues, in peer group supervision or reading groups."*

Group supervision is an essential learning experience. The interpersonal nature of these groups provides therapists an opportunity to navigate and manage relationships with other therapists. A good group supervision space also provides opportunity for therapists to express and explore their thoughts and feelings related to therapy patients and issues arising in session. No one therapist knows everything (nor are they expected to!); being in a group with therapists reinforces this notion and encourages vulnerability and openness to learning (Adams, 2024). Experiencing a diversity of opinions and views from other therapists in the group helps normalise concerns.

On a practical note, group supervision offers a good opportunity for supervisees to accrue supervision hours.

Peer supervision

Similar to group supervision, peer supervision comprises several therapists of the same general level of expertise and experience. It is a reciprocal peer arrangement, and not typically facilitated by any one member of the group.

Peer supervision involves discussion of ethical queries, patient presentations, and professional issues. It is an opportunity to discuss issues freely in a contained space in which confidentiality is assured. While typically scheduled for monthly meetings, peer supervision also promotes the opportunity for ad hoc and on-demand supervision at times when a timely or specific issue arises.

Peer supervision offers an invaluable support system. Many therapists are part of the same group for years or even decades, and hence they provide support through inevitable personal and professional challenges.

Specialist supervision

It is not possible for all supervision needs to be met by one supervisor. At times, specialist supervision will be required to obtain guidance or advice on a presentation or therapeutic modality beyond the remit of a supervisor.

A therapist's developmental needs may also be best served by having more than one supervisor at different stages of their training and career. An ethical and professional approach encourages clear communication around this from both parties; in the supervisory relationship, neither should feel they will cause offence or create a rupture by seeking additional supervision.

"Try out or use multiple supervisors. They will offer different things, so let yourself be stretched by different perspectives, feedback styles, and ways of working."

Self-supervision

Just as patients integrate the learnings from therapy, supervisees integrate knowledge from supervision. Over time, supervisees apply this knowledge without direct input from a supervisor. This may be regarding, for example, ethical decision-making or treatment planning.

Self-supervision does not preclude the need for ongoing external supervision, but it demonstrates the supervisee's advanced thinking and capacity for autonomous work. As a supervisor, it is especially pleasing to observe a supervisee reach a point of self-supervision; this creates space in the supervisory relationship to consider higher-order professional issues and more complex clinical queries.

Remedial supervision

In some instances, therapists are mandated to attend supervision by a regulatory body or licensing board. This typically follows a patient complaint, violation of ethical or professional obligation, or other egregious issue. The therapist is required to engage in specific supervision for a set duration regarding the complaint or issue.

These matters most often arise from dual relationships or multiple relationships with patients, insufficient record-keeping, and working outside of scope of competence. The most intriguing or shocking of these cases, such as therapists engaging in sexual relationships with patients, may reach the media or come to public attention, but ordinary matters that precipitate participation in remedial supervision are more mundane and represent the "slippery slope" behaviours that start as relatively benign and progress to being problematic, harmful, unethical, or, at worst, illegal (Barnett et al., 2014; Frankcom et al., 2016; Grenyer & Lewis, 2012).

Engaging in frequent and consistent supervision is a key strategy to avoid the ethical and professional pitfalls that may necessitate remedial supervision. Lack of engagement in supervision is a predictor of therapists being mandated to participate in remedial supervision. Prevention is always better than cure.

Selecting a supervisor

Supervisor selection is best considered as a "good fit" between supervisee and supervisor. This will be dependent on many dynamic factors, including emotional safety, availability, and congruence in personality and approach.

Several factors point to the selection of a good supervisor. Personal characteristics include resilience, humility, and openness to learning and feedback. Good supervisors show respect for supervisees and the profession. Contraindications to a good supervisory relationship include an exaggerated power differential (whether perceived or real), and either the supervisee or supervisor being fearful of negative personal or professional consequences of providing feedback (Denny et al., 2019).

"Find a good supervisor, someone whom you feel safe with and can share your worries with. I had the same person for supervision for eight years and it was the best thing I could do for my career as well as personal growth."

Good supervision is robust, supportive, non-blaming, unambiguous, and containing (Adams, 2024). A supervisory relationship in which the supervisee is not appropriately challenged may leave both parties feeling positive and content, but this is a false sense of confidence and is unlikely to foster ongoing learning and development.

A good supervisory relationship must feel safe. This includes active listening, empathy, encouragement, and respectful challenging. The supervisor must have the capacity to put the needs of the supervisee before their own, and be able to identify the supervisee's level of skill and knowledge and provide supervision and a supervisory relationship consistent with this (Adams, 2024; Frankcom et al., 2016).

It is unlikely that all supervisory needs will be met by one supervisor. Some supervisors may not be competent in a specific field (such as relationship counselling) or with a specific presentation or diagnosis (such as disordered eating). In such cases, the supervisee should seek additional specialist supervision outside of their primary supervisor relationship. This has become somewhat easier with the proliferation of video communication platforms (Barnett et al., 2014; White, 2001).

A preliminary 15-minute phone call or video chat with potential supervisors can be useful to initiate a supervisory relationship. A potential supervisor being too busy to take this call may be an indication that they will not be able to meet the needs of a supervisee, which often involves time outside sessions to review materials and documents.

Some questions to ask potential supervisors include:

- What is your therapeutic modality?
- What is your fee schedule? This includes policies around cancellation and charges for completing additional paperwork, such as for registration.
- What strategies do you use in supervision (i.e., role plays, video review, providing feedback on notes and reports)?
- What are your expectations around time frames for receiving material required for sessions, such as video/audio records and reports?
- In the instance of personal leave (whether planned or unexpected), do you have a colleague who is able to step in to provide supervision?
- Are there particular presentations or issues that you do not provide supervision about?

Develop a contract before supervision commences. Training organisations and professional bodies may provide a pro forma, with content dependent on the supervisees' training level and requirements around registration. Typically, supervision contracts include agreements around:

- Therapeutic modality
- Frequency and duration of sessions
- Modality (face-to-face, video)
- Fees, including cancellation fees, and person or organisation responsible for invoice payment
- Specific goals of supervision, usually framed in the language of SMART goals (Specific, Measurable, Achievable, Relevant, Time-based)
- Review dates for progress towards SMART goals

Being a supervisee

Supervision can only be as good as the supervisee allows. It is an opportunity for supervisees to hone skills, receive feedback, and develop as a therapist. Supervision is one of the only opportunities in which the focus is on the therapist, rather than the patient. Supervisees should be encouraged to embrace this opportunity for growth and development. Budget for the time and cost of supervision; consider it an essential investment in the lifelong learning of being a therapist.

Be prepared for supervision. Present an agenda at the start of each supervision session. If you are planning on seeking feedback on video or audio recordings, ensure the supervisor receives these with adequate time. Check with supervisors about their individual expectations of time frames for reviewing material and providing feedback.

Supervision is an opportunity for supervisees to demonstrate therapy skills and to indicate to the supervisor progress in both knowledge and skills. This also needs to be balanced with vulnerability and the demonstration of vulnerability and an openness to learning and integrating new knowledge. Supervisors who provide only positive feedback should be avoided; this collusion serves supervisees' egos but does little for learning.

All supervisory relationships inevitably come to an end. This may be after many years or a relatively short period of time. Terminating the relationship may be initiated by either party, perhaps due to a supervisor's retirement, or changing needs of a supervisee in terms of supervision around specific presentations or populations that are outside of the scope of the supervisor's area of knowledge or competence. It is hoped that this will be on good terms, but as with any relationship, supervisory relationships can also be difficult or sour over time. Communicating in a professional and courteous manner is always best in such situations, remembering that setting the foundations for reciprocal feedback early in the supervisory relationship is likely to assist during tricky times such as termination.

Being a supervisor

Supervision requires a different set of skills than therapy work. Overlap exists between the tasks of supervision and therapy, but competence as a therapist does not necessarily equate to being a good supervisor. In comparison to therapy, supervision entails greater maturity, comfort with authority, and nuanced evaluation. The essential tasks of therapy include offering support, promoting honesty, providing information, teaching skills, nurturing ethical judgment, assisting therapists with identify formation, and noticing and preventing burnout (McWilliams, 2021). Supervisors also have an important role in gate-keeping within the profession, including evaluation of trainees' competence in both knowledge and skills. Supervisors must also be alert and responsive to problematic ethical and professional behaviour of supervisees.

Similar to the provision of therapy, supervisors must be mindful of providing supervision that is within the scope of their knowledge and experience. Particular challenges that may arise within supervisory relationships include: the role of the supervisor, potential dual roles of providing personal therapy to supervisees and the amount and type of personal matters to be discussed during supervision, working with poorly performing supervisees, maintaining boundaries between provision of supervision and personal therapy (including amount of type of personal information shared by supervisees), and challenges with the supervisory alliance (McWilliams, 2021).

Accreditation requirements for supervisors differ between professionals and jurisdictions. Registration as a supervisor typically requires the therapist to have been in clinical practice for a set number of years. Supervisors generally complete a training course in supervision, together with ongoing supervision and continued professional development specifically related to supervision (Carroll, 2014).

Challenges in supervision

Just as in therapy with patients, difficulties can arise in supervision. Difficult supervisory experiences can undermine supervisees' confidence and can impact competence. The deleterious impact on supervisees' personal and professional sense of self also flows on to their work with patients.

Ideally, supervisory relationships should be reciprocal. Modern learning theories point to the benefit of bidirectional supervisory relationships, rather than the traditional unidirectional delivery of feedback from a learned elder to a novice learner. Feedback should be a shared two-way endeavour, in which supervisee and supervisor are attuned to and in step with each other. That is, the supervisor and supervisee should engage in mutual reflective evaluation of all aspects of supervision.

The power differential between parties in the supervisory relationship can result in reluctance from supervisees to engage in feedback dialogue. This is especially true in training programmes in which the supervisor may have a role in the supervisee's assessment or career trajectory. Reciprocal feedback can be facilitated by scheduling it as part of regular supervision, rather than an ad hoc arrangement or in response to difficulties within the therapeutic relationship (Denny et al., 2019).

"Seek supervision, the help of your trusted colleagues, and don't be fearful of letting others know when you're struggling."

The line between supervision and therapy can sometimes become blurred. The role of a supervisor will often include consideration of the supervisee's personal circumstances, particularly in therapeutic modalities such as psychodynamic or relationship psychotherapies. Personal disclosure can be helpful within the supervisory relationship; however, professional boundaries must always be maintained. The primary focus of supervision must be on patients; discussion of the supervisee's personal life should be contained to considerations of transference and countertransference. Always check in at the end of supervision to evaluate content covered and strategies discussed; if the focus continues to tip towards consideration of the supervisee's life and circumstances, both the supervisor and supervisee should work towards ensuring the supervisee is engaged in necessary personal therapy.

Personal therapy (be the patient)

Engaging in therapy as a patient represents the best way to learn about therapy.

---

*"You must have an experience of therapy yourself.
You need to know what it's like on the receiving end.
With all its vulnerability."*

Personal therapy is a compulsory element of training in some therapeutic modalities. Psychoanalytic training, for example, requires candidates to engage in several hours of personal therapy per week. Similar requirements exist in psychodynamic training. Training across other fields and across different jurisdictions may also include mandated personal therapy (Carlson, 2011).

Whether mandated or voluntary, all therapists are strongly encouraged to engage in personal therapy. The benefits of "being the patient" abound. Vicarious learning from an experienced therapist, modelling of skills (such as time management and reflective listening), and exposure to micro and macro skills, such as the use of specific phrases or strategies. A paradoxical effect may also occur – that is, as a patient, you may learn what *not* to do. A particular therapeutic style or skill may not resonate, and you may decide to not emulate it. This is all grist for the mill and represents essential learning experiences.

"Our ability to sit with uncertainty is a learnt skill, and one we cannot expect our clients to do if we can't do it for ourselves."

Most pertinently, personal therapy promotes reflection, self-awareness, and an understanding of the inextricable link between therapists' personal and professional selves (Hart, 1985). It provides an opportunity to identify and manage the processes unique to therapy, including the tendency to idealise therapy and therapists, feelings of dependence, and the experience of gratitude for the presence of a caring and attentive listener (Yalom, 2009). The therapist is their own most valuable tool; personal and professional experiences shape the therapist and their work, and therefore insight into the self is an essential aspect of professional competence. Engaging in personal therapy allows the therapist to mine the best source of data about patients – that is, our own feelings and interactions with the patient (Gabbard, 2005; Yalom, 2009).

The advantages of personal therapy for therapists have been long assumed. More recently, several studies have further articulated its usefulness; Rizq and Target (2008) describe it as a vehicle for genuine therapeutic engagement and a way for therapists to experience authentic emotional contact with themselves and others. Further, a study of seven therapists engaging in their own personal therapy identified several benefits for the therapists' own clinical work: orienting to the therapist (humanity, power, boundaries); orienting to the client (trust, respect, patience); and "listening with the third ear" (identifying the meeting with the unique needs of individual patients) (Macran et al., 1999).

> *"Get your own therapy! Regularly, and*
> *with people of varying modalities."*

Some therapists resist personal therapy. They may fear exposing their own vulnerabilities (to both themselves and the therapist), or they may worry that engaging in personal therapy would inadvertently reinforce a sense of imposter syndrome. Some buy into the false belief that therapists should and can fix their own problems (Arzt, 2020). On a practical note, therapy can be time-consuming and expensive. Like non-therapists, some therapists bemoan difficulty in finding the "right fit" in terms of therapists. None of these reasons are sufficient to neglect the need for personal therapy.

For various reasons, some therapists do not acknowledge the inevitable toll of working in a helping profession. Others deny (whether consciously or unconsciously) their difficult experiences, perhaps from shame of being afflicted by the same problems as their patients. Of course, therapists are humans too; just like patients, therapists experience personal crises and psychological distress (Denny, 2025; Gottlieb, 2022). But professional and applied knowledge of psychopathology and treatment of psychological distress do not provide immunity from personal troubles. Proper management is required to ensure therapists' own experiences do not adversely impact the capacity to perform all the tasks inherent to conducting therapy. All therapists require adequate support of the personal self, especially in times of personal hardship and psychological distress (Adams, 2024).

> *"Good supervision is key! Finding a good*
> *supervisor is as important as finding a good*
> *therapist! Which is also a good thing to do!"*

Self-exploration is a lifelong process (Rogers, 1961). Personal therapy is not a one-off task to be completed, but rather an ongoing undertaking that brings both professional and personal benefits.

Tips for therapists engaging in personal therapy:

- Engage with different therapists over time.
- Exercise patience in finding the "right" therapist.
- Ask colleagues for referrals to therapists. Some therapists do not advertise their services or availability, but are accessible through professional networks.
- Engage with different therapeutic modalities, including your own and any others that may pique your interest. This will likely change over time, with the evolution of your own personal and professional experiences and perspectives.
- Speak with candour and openness about your thoughts of being a therapist in therapy.
- Resist overlapping personal therapy with clinical supervision (Carroll, 2014).
- Consider the "best fit" for your stage of life and the concerns that come with it. Short-term behavioural therapy for concerns such as procrastination or insomnia might suit as some life stages, while deeper introspection through longer psychotherapy might suit at other times (Yalom, 2017).
- Reflect on your experiences of therapy, through journaling or other methods. Check in with yourself throughout the process of therapy – your capacity for vulnerability, experiences of transference and countertransference, and its impact on both your work as a therapist and your personal relationships and experiences (Kottler, 2010).

Professional development

Most registration and licensing boards stipulate requirements for hours of supervision and participation in continued professional development activities. This usually includes both formative and summative assessment (tasks which foster growth and reflection, and tasks with a formal assessment component). Professional boards may audit therapists to ensure completion of activities, recency of practice, and adequate hours of supervision and professional development. Often continued professional development includes an "active" component in which the participant must demonstrate their learnings and skills by participating in activities such as role plays or completing a written assessment or quiz.

Professional development may include readings, attending lectures and conferences, and participation in workshops. Therapists should develop an annual plan for continued professional development, including budget considerations (funds may be self-funded or allocated from an employer) and planning leave from work. Both of these usually need to be completed several months in advance.

"Research shows that five years after graduation, we have forgotten most of what we learned during our course. Do lots of professional development; when you come across one that really resonates for you, do it more than once, as there's no way we can remember it all or take it all in the first time."

In order to learn knowledge and skills in relation to specific patient presentations and patient populations, therapists are encouraged to engage in workshops given by expert clinicians in the field, preferably those who themselves continue to conduct clinical work (Fairburn, 2008). Therapists can keep updated about opportunities for workshops by registering their interest with specific training organisations and joining mailing lists of professional bodies who organise workshops and conferences.

Summary

- Supervision is a reciprocal relationship in which a more senior and experienced therapist offers oversight and training on clinical, ethical, and professional issues.
- Supervision is an integral activity for all therapists. It is particularly pertinent in the trainee and early-career stages but should be continued throughout a therapist's career.
- Types of supervision include individual, group, peer, specialist, and self. Mandated remedial supervision may also be indicated for therapists following an infringement or patient complaint.
- Good supervision is robust, supportive, non-blaming, unambiguous, and containing.
- Supervision can only be as good as the supervisee allows it to be. This requires preparation, insight, and active participation.
- Supervisory relationships should be reciprocal – that is, an exchange of feedback between supervisor and supervisee.

- Engaging in personal therapy is the best way to learn about therapy. Try different therapists and different therapeutic modalities over time.
- Continued professional development represents another part of supervision. This can include attending workshops, lectures, and seminars and completing readings.

Reference list

Adams, M. (2024). *The myth of the untroubled therapist* (2nd ed.). Routledge.

Arzt, N. (2020). *Sometimes therapy is awkward: A collection of life-changing insights for the modern clinician.* HMD Publishing.

Barnett, J. E., Zimmerman, J., & Walfish, S. (2014). *The ethics of private practice: A practical guide for mental health clinicians.* Oxford University Press.

Carlson, J. (2011). *Becoming a psychodynamic psychotherapist* [PhD thesis, Karolinska Institute].

Carroll, M. (2014). *Effective supervision for the helping professions* (2nd ed.). Sage Publications Ltd.

Corey, G., Corey, M. S., & Corey, C. (2024). *Issues & ethics in the helping professions* (11th ed.). Cengage.

Denny, B. (2025). *Talk to me: Lessons from patients and their therapist.* Routledge.

Denny, B., Brown, J., Kirby, C., Garth, B., Chesters, J., & Nestel, D. (2019). "I'm never going to change unless someone tells me I need to": Fostering feedback dialogue between GP supervisors and registrars. *Australian Journal of Primary Health, 25*(4), 374–379.

Fairburn, C. G. (2008). *Cognitive behavior therapy and eating disorders.* Guilford Press.

Frankcom, K., Stevens, B., & Watts, P. (2016). *Fit to practice.* Australian Academic Press.

Gabbard, G. O. (2005). *Psychodynamic psychiatry in clinical practice* (4th ed.). American Psychiatric Publications.

Gottlieb, L. (2022). *Maybe you should talk to someone: A therapist, her therapist, and our lives revealed.* Scribe Publications.

Grenyer, B. F., & Lewis, K. L. (2012). Prevalence, prediction, and prevention of psychologist m misconduct. *Australian Psychologist, 47*(2), 68–76. https://doi.org/10.1111/j.1742-9544.2010.00019.x

Hart, A. (1985, March). Becoming a psychotherapist: Issues of identity transformation. In *Issues in the training and development of psychotherapists.* Annual meeting of the Eastern Psychological Association.

Kottler, J. A. (2010). *On being a therapist* (4th ed.). Jossey-Bass.

Macran, S., Stiles, W., & Smith, J. (1999). How does personal therapy affect therapists' practice? *Journal of Counseling Psychology, 46*(4), 419–431.

McWilliams, N. (2011). *Psychoanalytic diagnosis*. Guilford Press.

McWilliams, N. (2021). *Psychoanalytic supervision*. Guilford Press.

Rizq, R., & Target, M. (2008). "The power of being seen": An interpretative phenomenological analysis of how experienced counselling psychologists describe the meaning and significance of personal therapy in clinical practice. *British Journal of Guidance & Counselling, 36*(2), 131–153. https://doi.org/10.1080/03069880801926418

Rogers, C. R. (1961). *On becoming a person: A therapist's view of psychotherapy*. Constable.

White, C. A. (2001). *Cognitive behaviour therapy for chronic medical problems: A guide to assessment and treatment in practice*. John Wiley.

Yalom, I. D. (2009). *The gift of therapy: Reflections on being a therapist*. Harper Perennial.

Yalom, I. D. (2017). *Becoming myself: A psychiatrist's memoir*. Scribe Publications.

The business of therapy **11**

"I'm looking forward to starting a quiet, peaceful, little private practice."

I have heard this statement or a variation of it from many trainee and early-career therapists. Some, having struggled with the fast pace and perceived complexity of presentations encountered during internships in hospitals or public mental health services, view private practice as a place of respite. Others say they are looking forward to autonomy and independence in their work. A subset of graduates launch into private practice with dollar signs in their eyes, viewing it as a lucrative opportunity after completing back-of-the-envelope calculations of high hourly rates and strong consumer demand (while neglecting or minimising expenses).

I reflected upon the idea of private practice being "quiet and peaceful" at the end of one of my own typical working weeks, detailed here:

Patient-related work included 20 therapy sessions and three supervision sessions. Notes were completed for each patient and supervision session. Correspondence was required for several patients, including letters to referrers and support letters for students requesting special accommodations for the upcoming exam period. Other tasks included a mandatory notification regarding safety concerns related to a child. I contacted a crisis service via phone (and was on hold for the better part of an hour) for a patient who presented to our session with clear and present suicidal ideation. I also responded to a subpoena (collating and sending a patient's file, after corresponding with the judicial registrar regarding redaction of information that I deemed irrelevant to the court matter). Late one evening, I received a one-line email from a new patient, long estranged from their family: "My dad died".

DOI: 10.4324/9781003533030-11

I also participated in my own therapy and supervision sessions and attended a full-day professional development workshop. Each required time away from clinical work. By virtue of being self-employed, these activities were all self-funded.

Business-related tasks included following up an overdue patient invoice, paying for professional indemnity insurance renewal, organising and lodging my quarterly tax statement, and negotiating with the owner of our consulting rooms regarding a property maintenance issue. Last, I updated my professional will (a document stating business arrangements and plans for patient care, in case of my death or incapacitation) to include a new nominee.

Like many therapists, I also juggle parenting responsibilities and home tasks, and I endeavour to maintain self-care and enjoy some version of leisure activity.

Quiet and peaceful? I think not.

★★

Therapy offers the opportunity for a long and prosperous career. Its largely sedentary nature means that most therapists can work in some capacity beyond usual retirement age. Diversification of skills and roles beyond the provision of therapy is also possible, with therapists in high demand for therapy-adjacent positions, such as supervision and teaching.

Private practice represents just one setting of many in which therapists can work. To this end, trainee and early-career therapists are urged to think broadly about career prospects and resist the temptation to enter straight into a private setting. The entire business of the trainee and early-career stages of being a therapist is to learn therapy skills. This is an opportune time to work in an environment in which learning and support is facilitated, without unnecessary worry about operating a business.

I will belabour this point time and time again. However, personal and professional experience tells me that the business and financial aspects of being a therapist are an omnipresent concern for some therapists, often thought of long before the ink on registration paperwork is dry. Would-be private therapists may be attracted by financial aspirations, opportunity for autonomy, and flexibility of work arrangements. But the potential benefits of private practice or running a therapy clinic should be considered together with its inherent challenges.

Many therapists aspire to work in a private practice setting. Despite this, business and managerial aspects of operating a therapy practice are not typically included in training courses. This is often the focus of criticism from early-career therapists who aspire to work in a private practice setting. However, solid knowledge and skills around therapy are a necessary precursor to learning business practices.

"In your early career, work in the public system to become skilled and confident with risk assessment and management, and to ensure you have a solid understanding of how the public health system works."

The image of a therapist perpetuated in popular culture – think Dr Jennifer Melfi from _The Sopranos_ or the boundary-crossing Paul Weston from _In Treatment_ – shows a therapist working in some form of private practice (Gabbard, 2002). The therapist depicted on the screen – typically a serene, cardigan-wearing individual sitting on a comfortable sofa in a warmly lit consulting room – gives a superficial (and often inaccurate) representation of a therapist working in private practice.

In some countries, such as Australia, government rebates or insurance coverage applies to therapy services. Rebates and insurance coverage may reduce the out-of-pocket cost of therapy, making it an increasingly popular choice for patients seeking treatment. This incentive has precipitated a change in the therapy landscape; private practice was traditionally viewed as reserved for very experienced therapists who had "earned their stripes" in other mental health services such as public hospitals. However, there is now a sharp increase in graduates entering private practice directly from University or other training programmes (Frankcom et al., 2016). Private practice is less common in countries such as the United Kingdom, where typically only very experienced therapists enter into private work. In the United States, private therapy practices are often contingent on patients' insurance arrangements. Licensing and practice requirements differ between jurisdictions.

Regardless of these differences, many considerations are common across all private practice settings.

Private practice

Therapists can hang their shingle and commence private practice, typically without needing a special license or any specific permit.[1] However, this does not mean all therapists are best suited to private practice, particularly in the early-career stage.

Private practice comes without many of the benefits inherent to working in an organisation: sick leave, carers' leave, insurance coverage, retirement fund contributions, provisions for supervision, professional development activities (via stipend or direct payment), and professional oversight by senior clinicians. Moreover, the connection with other therapists and professionals, whether through formal mentorship or informal "corridor conversations", is largely absent from private practice settings. The vicarious learning that comes from observation of experienced therapists cannot usually be replicated in private practice. These collegial activities are most valuable to trainee and early-career therapists.

Private practice can be a rewarding and profitable enterprise. It undoubtedly has perks. This is particularly true for therapists who are self-motivated, financially savvy, organised, skilled with time management, administratively minded, and who enjoy working independently and having autonomy over their own work. Robust business skills may be innate for some, or they may be aided by professional development or additional training specific to business considerations.

On the flip side, I have seen more than a few therapists leave private practice feeling dejected, exhausted, financially depleted, and emotionally demoralised. Just like any small business, running a therapy business can present financial challenges, particularly in the first few years of operation.

The burden of patient complaints – which are more frequent in private practice in comparison to other therapy settings – can have moral, legal, financial, and licensing ramifications. Sadly, therapists who have experienced such difficulties sometimes leave the professional entirely. With confidence battered and competence queried, some therapists generalise their negative experiences to all therapy settings. This is a loss not only for the individual therapist, but for the broader community and health-care services in which therapists are highly valued and much-needed.

Therapists need to consider their stage of life and capacity to work the hours required to fulfil the ethical and clinical responsibilities of private practice. Demand for out-of-hours and weekend appointments is typically strong; having young children or other family responsibilities may make meeting this demand difficult, which in turn can impact the financial viability and sustainability of private practice.

Therapists in private practice often have the capacity to set their own work hours and maintain flexibility for attending personal and professional appointments. However, the reality remains that sessions must be booked, and patients need to be seen, for a therapist to derive an income from working in private practice. The notion of flexibility is twofold; therapists in private practice can enjoy a flexible work schedule, but this may also extend to working unsociable hours or making other sacrifices with time.

Ethics of private practice

In comparison to their colleagues in organisational settings, therapists in private practice are at increased risk of being the subject of a patient complaint. In an average 30-year career, approximately 20% of therapists will have a complaint or notification lodged against them (Frankcom et al., 2016). Statistics from Australia and South Africa, respectively, indicate approximately 0.6% of complaints to be upheld, resulting in disciplinary action from licensing and registration boards (Grenyer & Lewis, 2012; Nortje & Hoffman, 2015). These figures clearly indicate that being the subject of a complaint does not necessarily indicate wrongdoing on behalf of the therapist. However, regardless of whether a complaint is upheld, the notification and investigation processes represent an unpleasant and often avoidable professional and personal experience. To this end, therapists working in private practice must be especially mindful of compliance with ethical and professional regulations. Therapists must protect themselves against ill-informed or vexatious claims, while also respecting clients' opinions and positions.

Therapists in private practice have a measure of professional privilege. There is often no immediate or direct oversight of their work. This autonomy may be misconstrued by some as permission to take shortcuts or work to a lower standard. Consequences for ethical transgressions and professional violations are usually delayed; reporting and investigation processes are slow-moving behemoths, often taking many months or, in some cases, years. Behavioural principles (with which all therapists should be familiar) indicate that distal or delayed consequences provide less deterrent in comparison to immediate sanctions or reprimand. Hence, the autonomy and self-regulation common to private practice provides an environment in which ethical transgressions may go unnoticed or not attended to.

Organisational workplaces provide greater measures and safeguards against ethical and professional transgressions and the reporting of these. Internal investigations may result in complaints being resolved prior to referral to registration or licensing boards. This provides a "third party" perspective and overview of therapists' work. Some aspects of organisational structures (direct supervision, management, collegial peer relationships) that provide these safeguards are absent in private practice. This arguably leaves the therapist vulnerable to practising in an unethical or unprofessional manner, whether knowingly or unknowingly. All therapists have blind spots; working within an organisational structure may assist in identifying and managing these before they lead to ethical transgressions or professional misdemeanours.

Complaints against therapists in private practice typically reflect problematic professional behaviour across several key areas (Barnett et al., 2014; Frankcom et al., 2016; Nortje & Hoffman, 2015):

- Qualifications and licensing (false or misleading advertising or marketing about training and skills, misuse of protected titles)
- Boundary violations (dual relationships, sexual relationships)
- Poor communication (regarding fees, course/length of treatment, expectations of therapeutic outcomes; informed consent)
- Lack of clarity around fees, and financial policies and procedures
- Inadequate supervision and/or lack of continued professional development
- Insufficient note-taking and record-keeping
- Competence (including negligence, practising outside of scope, continued treatment of non-improving or deteriorating patient)
- Poor or mismanaged business practices (including insurance fraud)

By its very nature, private practice can be isolating. Contact with other therapists may be few and far between. Even with shared consulting rooms or shared reception/administration, therapists in these settings are often "ships in the night" – aware of each other's presence but often denied the opportunity for conversation and collaboration due to time constraints.

"Avoid burnout through developing good-quality professional networks (formal and informal), self-care, and ensuring you can 'switch off' from work."

Therapists working in private practice often find themselves experiencing a unique kind of exhaustion at the end of the workday. Understandably, their "social battery" is depleted after hours of focusing on patients and their needs. Yet, given the lack of reciprocity in therapeutic relationships, their own need for affiliation has often not been met. Thus, the paradox of being a therapist – after a whole day of listening and talking, many therapists do not wish to engage in further conversation. This can lend itself to social isolation and lack of engagement in leisure activities. In turn, this is a clear and consistent precursor to the therapist experiencing burnout (see Chapter 10).

Practising alone need not mean practising in isolation. Therapists working in private practice will benefit from pre-emptively organising peer supervision and professional connections. This may be with therapists working from the same location, or with others who have similar professional interests. Maintaining these connections not only reduces the risk of isolation and burnout, but it will go some way to providing checks and balances around ethical and professional behaviour for solo therapists.

"Go slowly. Pace yourself."

Working in private practice

Several structures exist for working in private practice. These differ across professions and jurisdictions. Laws around employment, taxation, and business structures need to be considered for each.

Sole private practice

A sole private practice is a one-person therapy business. Typically, the therapist runs all aspects of the private practice. The therapist works independently and maintains their own patient load and responsibility for bookings, notes, and billing. A therapist in sole private practice usually rents a consulting room by the day or week or may work from a home office.

Some therapists may group together to share rooms and other resources, such as administrative assistance. In this case, therapists generally maintain independence over their own work conditions, but they can enjoy the benefits of shared costs and a collegial workplace.

Subcontractors

This is a popular option for early-career therapists. Subcontracting represents a good option to commence private practice in an environment which (hopefully) allows the therapist to focus on clinical work while administration tasks and practice overheads are managed.

Various models exist for subcontracting of therapy services. Generally, the company or organisation to whom the therapist is contracted provides administrative support, referrals, a consulting room, and access to resources such as psychometric testing materials. Subcontractors pay an agreed-upon fee, which is usually based on percentage of fees earned. This can vary from 20% to 50% (or more) depending on the specific provisions of administrative and other support.

The subcontractor therapist remains independent in their work and should be free to set their own hours and make independent choices around patient load and number of sessions worked. Formal supervision is not typically included, nor are items such as computers or stationery.

Employees

Employees work under employment contracts. In comparison to subcontracting and sole practice, employment is typically more structured in terms of set hours, consistent wages, benefits, and leave. Some form of supervision is usually included, in addition to tools and materials required to provide therapy services.

Being the boss – employing or subcontracting other therapists

Managing a team of subcontractors or employees can be financially rewarding, but it comes with a heavy workload. Some senior therapists thrive in this role – mentoring therapists, working through business models and decision-making, hiring and training staff. However, many report reduced opportunity to conduct their own clinical work, as much of their time becomes consumed by business considerations. De-skilling is a risk here.

Staff retention is a common challenge in employing or subcontracting therapists. Competent therapists are likely to eventually depart to start their own private practice, leaving a revolving door of therapists who require induction, training, and ongoing supervision and management. Rapid staff turnover is not typically conducive to good therapeutic care; patients and referrers may vote with their feet and look for a therapist with whom they are able to have a more stable therapeutic relationship.

Running a therapy business

Patient care must be paramount in a private practice. But private practice is also a business from which the therapist derives their income. These are not

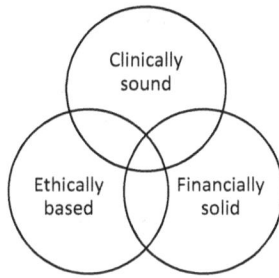

Figure 11.1 Successful private practice is informed by three broad components.

mutually exclusive concepts, but they can easily come into conflict. Each requires careful consideration and ongoing management.

Three key factors contribute to success in private practice. Balancing these three components takes a broad skill set, in addition to an ability to quickly shift between clinical, ethical, and financial obligations (see Figure 11.1).

These factors may seem diametrically opposed. Rarely will the three align with ease, even for the most skilled and experienced therapist. Concurrent confidence and competence across these areas – being clinically sound, ethically based, and financially solid – requires skill, tenacity, insight, and business acumen. Like most ventures, a modicum of good fortune along the way also helps.

Financial considerations

Therapists often have a complicated relationship with money. This is particularly true for trainee and early-career therapists, who may have become accustomed to working without pay or with minimal pay during training and internships in the early years of training and work. To some, therapy is assumed to be altruistic service, and therefore collecting fees for the provision of care seems counterintuitive (Adams, 2024). This may be especially true with patients experiencing financial hardship, whether that hardship is real or perceived by either the therapist or the patient (Barnett et al., 2014). It may seem emotionally unfathomable to earn an income for a job from which such fascination and satisfaction is derived (McWilliams, 1999).

Therapy is not coffee with a friend. Therapists are trained professionals, and their time and expertise must be adequately compensated. Self-abrogation about money is not compatible with sustaining a private practice. The provision of ongoing therapeutic care for patients requires the therapist to be remunerated.

Nancy McWilliams (2011) offers a neat script for responding to patients' queries about charging fees for therapy services. Her style is unapologetic and direct:

> I charge what I do because this is how I earn a living, helping people with emotional problems.
>
> (p. 77)

In private practice, time is money. It is imperative for each therapist to construct a budget, based on their unique circumstances, and financial expectations and responsibilities.

Figure 11.2 shows a basic formula for working as a therapist in private practice. These factors can be entered into a spreadsheet and used to calculate private practice income. Each variable can be adjusted to derive the necessary number of sessions, fees, and days of work required to meet desired take-home pay.

With a high hourly fee, private practice is typically thought to be a lucrative endeavour. Many therapists new to private practice are initially impressed by their financial position, before realising expenses and taxes have not been properly accounted for. Many are surprised by a hefty tax bill at the end of their first year in private practice, especially for those who have transitioned from roles in which taxes and other costs have been managed by employers.

Frequent (i.e., weekly) reconciliation of income and outgoings is a necessary process for therapists working in private practice. A simple strategy here is to allocate funds into three accounts, with equal thirds allocated to personal pay, expenses, and taxation. It is better to overestimate expenses and tax payments than to owe amounts on either.

Each therapist will have unique business expenses. This will be based on patient population, therapeutic modality, and professional and personal preferences. Common private practice expenses are outlined in Table 11.1. This list is non-exhaustive. Cost estimates and dollar figures have not been included, as these change over time and vary greatly.

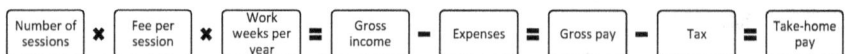

Number of sessions $\times$ Fee per session $\times$ Work weeks per year $=$ Gross income $-$ Expenses $=$ Gross pay $-$ Tax $=$ Take-home pay

Figure 11.2 Basic formula for calculating private practice income.

Table 11.1 Typical expenses incurred for therapists in private practice.

Category	Expense
Office	Consulting room hire (daily, weekly, or annual)
	Administrative support/secretarial services
	Stationery
	Copy/print/scan machine
	Filing cabinets or other storage space for files
	Credit card facility
Patient-related	Psychometric measures
	Assessment test kits
	Equipment (e.g., fidget toys, arts and crafts supplies, EMDR lightbar, workbooks, patient handouts)
Professional services	Accounting
	Banking
	Supervision
	Legal representation
	Professional indemnity insurance
Technology	Computer
	Internet connection
	Software (practice management; accounting/billing)
	Website – design, hosting, renewal
	Printer/copier/scanner
Communication	Telephone
	Telehealth or video platform subscription
	Fax/eFax service
	Postage
Professional registration and affiliations	Licensing/registration fees

(Continued)

Table 11.1 (Continued)

Category	Expense
	Association membership
Financial planning	Contribution to superannuation/retirement fund
	Student debt payments
Professional development	Workshops
	Conferences
	Supervision
	Books/literature

Fee schedules

Money is often a taboo subject for therapists. This is especially true for trainee and early-career therapists, who during years of study and training have likely worked on a voluntary basis or for a reduced fee. Many people, including therapists, who train and work within a helping profession are not primarily motivated by money (Adams, 2024).

It is common to grapple with the notion of charging fees for service. But few therapists – particularly at an early-career stage – can afford to work for free. Nor should they. Student debt, years of training, and loss of earnings during study and unpaid internships can lead to a sense of learned helplessness around fees.

Sigmund Freud, perhaps the best-known therapist to have ever worked in private practice, espoused payment for treatment to be essential. Freud linked better therapeutic outcomes with the financial investment made by patients, noting payment diminished some of the patient's resistance to therapy. He viewed payment as an indication of the patient's willingness to delve into deeper psychological terrain. The utility of fees was upheld by later research, in which open dialogue about fees is associated with enhanced psychotherapy outcomes (Pasternack, 1988), and patients' increased expectations of themselves and their therapist in the therapeutic process (Yoken & Berman, 1984). More recent research conducted in community and student clinics, however, has demonstrated fees to have no impact on therapeutic gains (Clark & Kimberly, 2014; De Beurs et al., 2018).

It is important for early-career therapists to adopt a professional approach to setting and charging fees for therapy. Just like therapy itself, consistency and clear communication around business arrangements and fees is key. This provides containment for the patient and therapist. Transparency around fees can help inform patients and also reduces administrative burden associated with responding to queries via phone and email regarding fees. This may include fee schedules and fee policies being listed on a therapist's website and other professional service directories.

Fees should be stated in writing and agreed upon by patients by way of a signed document. This may be included on the patient intake form, together with demographic information and personal details. Agreement to fee policy should outline session fees, cancellation and "no show" charges, and debt collection. This represents an important aspect of informed consent (see Chapter 2). With a considerable percentage of complaints to regulatory bodies and licensing boards focused on fees and business practices, transparency in this area may help prevent misunderstandings or formal complaints (Barnett et al., 2014; Frankcom et al., 2016).

It is useful for therapists to create a set script around fee schedules and fee policies. This can be used both written and verbal communication. Information regarding insurance or other applicable rebates should also be included. Be clear and direct, and always ask if patients have any queries regarding fees.

> The fee per session is X. Fees are payable on the day of service, via cash or credit card. The charge for non-attendance is Y, and the charge for late cancellation is Z.

Setting a fee schedule

A fee schedule refers to a list of fees. Some therapists or clinics adopt one fee for all patients, while others may offer concession fees for some patients, including students, low-income earners, or aged pensioners.

Therapists in private practice generally have autonomy in setting their own fees. It is the decision of patients to accept the service at an agreed-upon rate. Fee schedules set by therapists will be impacted by many factors, including years of experience, niche area or expertise, therapeutic modality, demand for services, demographic and socio-economic characteristics of patients, and overhead costs (consulting room rental, administration support, insurance, etc.).

Therapists must be mindful of not taking financial advantage of current or potential patients, some of whom may be vulnerable or have impaired decision-making due to acute or chronic psychological distress.

Scheduled fees may be set by insurers or third-party payers. In these instances, it may be unlawful to prescribe alternative fees, or to charge patients attending through an insurer or third-party a "gap fee" (the difference between the therapist's fee and the scheduled fee set by the insurer or third party).

There is no right or wrong approach to setting fees, nor any magic dollar amount which should be charged per session. Many professional associations publish annual fee guidelines, calculated to reflect inflation and other financial considerations. Therapists should work towards identifying a fee structure consistent with their values, without underselling themselves or their skills. It may take time and a few iterations to settle upon a fee structure that strikes a balance between not leaving the therapist vulnerable to financial hardship while also matching the needs of patients.

Given the nature of therapy work, money can become a process issue. That is, it can contribute to or interfere with the therapeutic relationship and may therefore have implications for treatment and treatment outcomes. Consistency with fees and policies helps patients to feel contained and allows the therapist to focus on the true business of therapy without unnecessary distraction – that is, therapeutic treatment.

Fee reductions and pro-bono work

Providing pro-bono or reduced-fee services can benefit patients and also be rewarding for therapists. However, it may also foster feelings of resentment for therapists. Most therapists have a variation of the story in which a fee reduction is negotiated with a patient on the basis of financial hardship, only to have said patient advise a few weeks later of their plans for an upcoming overseas holiday, extended vacation, or home renovations. It is difficult for even the most generous and open-minded therapist to resist negative feelings in this situation. Like any interpersonal relationship, resentment in the therapeutic dynamic can be a toxic rupture that requires skilled repair. Ruptures resulting from issues around fees can be minimised and managed with appropriate and timely planning. Avoid having money become the battleground for other, less articulated struggles (McWilliams, 1999).

Carefully consider when and if concession or reduced fees are offered. Definitions of wealth and poverty and ideas about the who and why of applying pro-bono and concession fees also vary widely. I do not endorse the approach of dissecting patients' tax returns or financial situation to decipher the affordability of therapy for individual patients (Cozolino, 2004), preferring instead to take the view that patients choose how and where they spend their money. Patients who cannot or will not meet your fee schedules can be referred elsewhere; other referral options exist.

Negotiations around fees will depend on several factors, including therapeutic modality and patient need. Some therapists who practise therapies that require patients to attend several times per week, such as psychoanalysis, offer a reduced rate to incentivise attendance.

Reviewing and revising fees

Fees must be revised and reviewed regularly in order to run a private practice that is viable and sustainable. Many a therapist has found themselves in a financially difficult position due to reluctance to increase fees in a manner consistent with inflation and other costs. Reviewing and revising fees should be a regular activity, either yearly or half-yearly, at the beginning of the calendar or financial year. Therapists in private practice can be guided by recommended fee schedules from their professional bodies or associations, which are typically updated annually.

In general, therapists seem to fret more than patients over incremental fee increases. This is a countertransference issue and should be taken to supervision (i.e., the therapist may be concerned that they are not delivering therapy to a standard that deserves better remuneration).

Once a fee is set, maintain consistency for a reasonable period of time. Unexpected and frequent changes to fees can be destabilising and unsettling for patients. This is arguably unethical and unprofessional, and it is likely to be disruptive and destabilising to therapeutic rapport.

Fee changes should always be communicated to patients in writing. Email or letter is sufficient. A notice in the waiting area may be overlooked or disregarded. Keep the correspondence regarding fees short and factual. Invite patients to make contact with any queries or concerns. There is no need to justify the specifics around fee increases, such as whether they are necessitated by increased costs or overheads borne by the therapist or the clinic. This information is not relevant for patients and blurs the lines between therapy and business processes. Again, this can be disruptive to therapeutic rapport.

Cancellation and non-attendance fees

From both a therapeutic and business perspective, it is necessary to enforce cancellation and non-attendance fees (with the exception of instances of genuine ill health).

Always check in on patients who do not attend a session, and always keep a note in your records of your attempts to reach them. Fairburn (2008) recommends contacting the patient 15 minutes following the scheduled appointment time, expressing concern for their absence and offering to reschedule the appointment.

It is the business practice of some therapists and clinics to store patients' credit cards on file, and to charge automatically in instances of late cancellation or missed appointment. A colleague's recent experience reiterated my stances against this. The patient, usually reliable and punctual, did not attend a scheduled telehealth session. Several days later, my colleague was notified of the patient's death. Imagine, for a moment, justifying an automatic non-attendance fee to a family member or during a coronial inquest. This is a notable example of the need to prioritise patient care in all aspects of business and fee arrangements.

Managing debts

Some patients will violate the therapeutic contract by not paying fees as agreed.

Prudent therapists collect fees on the day of service (or as close to the day of service as possible). Think behavioural principles here – the recency effect tells us that current matters are in the forefront of the mind, while proximal or distal events soon drop down the list of priorities. The same is true of an invoice or bill with a long lead time until its due date.

Therapists tend to tie themselves in knots about the specifics and perceived peculiarities of any one outstanding fee. Having money owed can precipitate feelings of resentment, anger, and disappointment. A clear, pre-emptive policy around debt collection can help alleviate some of these problems. This should be included as part of informed consent prior to the patient engaging in therapy. Chasing debt is an unenviable task and is unfortunately unavoidable for most businesses, including therapists and clinics. Referring to a clear policy which has been sighted and signed by the patient is one way to minimise these problems.

Therapeutic modality also plays a role in managing patient debts. In order to avoid "corridor conversations" and to maintain a therapeutic rather than administrative relationship, some therapists use remote billing practices such as emailing invoices or using online credit card payment services to collect fees. This helps contain time with patients to the consulting room, avoiding any clinical information being discussed in the waiting room or other shared areas.

In case of outstanding fees, direct communication is best:

> I've noticed payment for your sessions is often late. This means a late fee is applied. To avoid this and to ensure we can continue our work together without disruption, I am going to suggest an alternative payment method for future sessions. This could include collecting your credit card details for automatic processing of session fees, or you bringing cash to our sessions. Which would best suit you?

Perhaps with the exception of therapists who conduct assessments and those who prepare lengthy reports, debts in private practice do not usually extend to an amount suitable for litigation or referral to a debt collection agency.

Contingency planning

Therapists in private practice need to ensure provisions are made for life's events, both foreseeable and unforeseeable. This includes but is not limited to death, incapacitation, illness (transient or serious, physical or psychological), and times during which leave will be required to care for family members or loved ones.

Financial arrangements include retirement planning, financial planning, insurance, provisions for sick leave and vacation, student loan repayments, and taxes. Private practice brings variable income from day to day, week to week, month to month, and year to year. Holiday season and personal leave – both typically expensive times – also impacts income and cashflow. This necessitates the adoption of different financial habits in comparison to therapists working for organisations where a regular wage is issued, in addition to benefits covering vacation leave, sick leave, health insurance, and other contingencies.

Therapists in private practice are particularly vulnerable to financial concerns and economic downturn (Adams, 2024). Therapy may be deemed a luxury by some, and it is therefore an expense culled when household purse strings are tightened during difficult economic times. Therapists who provide treatment funded by insurers or government-supported payment schemes also remain susceptible to changes in legislation and funding.

'Til death do us part

Many therapists tend to avoid existential matters and seem in a state of denial about their own mortality (Yalom, 2008). This is despite the introspective nature inherent to working as a therapist and the role of therapists in discussing and considering difficult matters, such as unexpected life transitions and death. But death will come to us all, and incapacitation will impact some. All therapists have an ethical and professional responsibility to prepare for death and incapacitation.

The death or incapacitation of a therapist can have serious implications for patients. Therapists must make provisions for the care of clients and provide instructions for appropriate processes around records in the event of their death or incapacitation. Similar in structure to a personal will, a practice contingency plan outlines arrangements regarding office access, patient care, record-keeping, insurance and registration details, managing outstanding income and debts, and other business considerations. Arrangements should be stated for notifying current patients of the circumstances surrounding your absence, keeping in mind the type and amount of information with which you are comfortable with patients being informed (American Psychological Association, 2014; Australian Psychological Society, 2021).

Executors or nominees are drawn from colleagues within the same profession. Unlike a personal will, it is not appropriate for family members of friends to be appointed. The role is best filled by a trusted colleague with whom the therapist shares a professional understanding but not a close personal acquaintance, as their ability to carry out necessary tasks (particularly communicating with patients) may be impacted by an emotional response to the therapist's death or incapacitation.

A final word on private practice

Therapy is a highly sought-after profession. Employment opportunities abound. While popular, private practice represents only one area of work. Therapists are well-placed to use skills in a variety of employment settings.

Early-career therapists are encouraged to take the opportunity to try different areas of practice and employment settings. These may include schools, community health services, forensic work (prison, judicial system), academia (teaching, tutor roles), research (research assistant, trial administration), residential care, child protection services, case management, hospitals, disability work, youth work, rehabilitation settings, and human relations. These are just a few of the career options available to therapists. Each typically provide employment security, steady income, and the opportunity to work within a team.

"Most trainee and early-career therapists would benefit from at least two to three years in hospital-based, community, or government roles. Entering straight into private practice does not best serve therapists or patients."

Whatever your approach to private practice, start low and go slow. Private practice can be commenced while working a substantive role with an organisation. Some therapists choose to maintain this balance in perpetuity, as it provides balance, security, and flexibility.

Do not put all your eggs in the private practice basket too quickly or without a fall-back plan. It will take time to find a niche, build a caseload, and determine the business processes and procedures consistent best suited to your skill set and values.

Summary

- Trainee and early-career therapists should ideally focus on acquisition and mastery of skills. Focusing too heavily on business aspects of therapy can detract from attaining and practising these essential skills.
- Early-career therapists benefit from the structure and processes afforded by working with an organisation. This includes supervision, sick leave, and consistent income.
- Private practice provides a long-term career option for therapists. Its sedentary nature and flexible work model mean many therapists can work beyond typical retirement age.
- Therapists in private practice enjoy professional privilege, including autonomous decision-making and flexible work hours. This should not be mistaken for permission to cut corners or practise at a subpar level.

- All therapists must maintain practice that is clinically sound and ethically based. Therapists in private practice have the added responsibility of maintaining a practice that is financially solid.
- Challenges associated with private practice include maintaining professional boundaries and managing finances and other business considerations.
- Therapists in private practice are at higher risk of committing ethical and professional transgressions. They are more frequently the subject of patient complaints and disciplinary action.
- Contingency planning is an important aspect of ensuring appropriate patient care in the instance of the therapist's unexpected death or incapacitation. A professional will can be used to set stipulations for aspects of patient care to be carried out by an appropriate person. This includes notes, records, communication, and, in some instances, ongoing provision of therapy.

Note

1 Licensing requirements and eligibility for different employment settings vary by jurisdiction.

Reference list

Adams, M. (2024). *The myth of the untroubled therapist* (2nd ed.). Routledge.

American Psychological Association. (2014). *Your professional will: Why and how to create.* https://www.apaservices.org/practice/good-practice/professional-will-instructions.pdf

Australian Psychological Society. (2021). Understanding practice contingency plans. *InPsych, 43*(3).

Barnett, J. E., Zimmerman, J., & Walfish, S. (2014). *The ethics of private practice: A practical guide for mental health clinicians.* Oxford University Press.

Clark, P., & Kimberly, C. (2014). Impact of fees among low-income clients in a training clinic. *Contemporary Family Therapy, 36*(3), 363–368. https://doi.org/10.1007/s10591-014-9303-9

Cozolino, L. (2004). *The making of a therapist.* Norton.

De Beurs, E., Warmerdam, E. H., Oudejans, S. C. C., Spits, M., Dingemanse, P., De Graaf, S. D. D., De Groot, I. W., Houben, H., Kuyck, W. G. E., Noorthoorn, E. O., Nugter, M. A., Robbers, S. C. C., & Van Son, G. E. (2018). Treatment outcome, duration, and costs: A comparison of performance indicators using data from eight mental health care providers in The Netherlands. *Administration and Policy in Mental Health and Mental Health Services Research, 45*(2), 212–223. https://doi.org/10.1007/s10488-017-0818-x

Fairburn, C. G. (2008). *Cognitive behavior therapy and eating disorders*. Guilford Press.

Frankcom, K., Stevens, B., & Watts, P. (2016). *Fit to practice*. Australian Academic Press.

Gabbard, G. O. (2002). *The psychology of the sopranos: Love, death, desire, and betrayal in America's favourite gangster family*. Basic Books.

Grenyer, B. F., & Lewis, K. L. (2012). Prevalence, prediction, and prevention of psychologist misconduct. *Australian Psychologist, 47*(2), 68–76. https://doi.org/10.1111/j.1742-9544.2010.00019.x

McWilliams, N. (1999). *Psychoanalytical case formulation*. Guilford Press.

McWilliams, N. (2011). *Psychoanalytic diagnosis*. Guilford Press.

Nortje, N., & Hoffman, W. A. (2015). Ethical misconduct by registered psychologists in South Africa during the period 2007–2013. *South African Journal of Psychology, 45*(2), 260–270.

Pasternack, S. A. (1988). The clinical management of fees during psychotherapy and psychoanalysis. *Psychiatric Annals, 18*(2), 112–117. https://doi.org/10.3928/0048-5713-19880201-13

Yalom, I. D. (2008). *Staring at the sun: Overcoming the terror of death*. Scribe Publications.

Yoken, C., & Berman, J. S. (1984). Does paying a fee for psychotherapy alter the effectiveness of treatment? *Journal of Consulting and Clinical Psychology, 52*(2), 254–260. https://doi.org/10.1037/0022-006X.52.2.254

Index

For Product Safety Concerns and Information please contact our EU
representative GPSR@taylorandfrancis.com
Taylor & Francis Verlag GmbH, Kaufingerstraße 24, 80331 München, Germany

www.ingramcontent.com/pod-product-compliance
Lightning Source LLC
Chambersburg PA
CBHW052002270326
41929CB00015B/2758